Men's Herbs and Hormonal Health

Testosterone, BPH, Alopecia, Adaptogens, Prostate Health, and Much More

By Joey Lott

www.joeylotthealth.com

Publishing services provided by **Archangel Ink**

ISBN: 1518666868
ISBN-13: 978-1518666865

Table of Contents

Why Metabolism, Hormones, and Herbs 5

Some Definitions 11

Hormonal Health 14

Inflammation 15

Immunity 17

Metabolism 19

Thyroid 27

Sex Hormones 48

Reducing Chronic Inflammation 60

Immune Modulation 65

Sleep 68

Stress 73

Prostate and Urinary Health 77

Hair Health 89

Insulin 96

Antibacterial Herbs 100

Liver 104

Sex 110

A Man's Herbal Guide 115

Conclusion 143

Resources 144

Get My Future Books FREE 150

Connect With Me 151

One Small Favor 152

About the Author 153

Why Metabolism, Hormones, and Herbs

This is a book about the connections between metabolism, stress, herbs, and other lifestyle choices. I believe that what is offered here in this book is truly unique and valuable. This is a book about men's herbs, but it is so much more as well. Rather than trying to give you some generic list of herbs, actions, and properties, I hope to offer you a practical, personal guide to discovering ways to experience vibrant health that includes using herbs, but certainly isn't limited to herbs.

What you'll find is that I am fairly non-dogmatic about most things, and I take an approach that is largely inclusive rather than restrictive. I do have opinions, and I am not afraid to state them. However, I try to keep it simple and share what I have actually experienced, rather than what sounds nice ideologically.

To that end, I do not espouse a restrictive diet or lifestyle. I have tried restrictive diets and lifestyles over the years with disastrous results. And, as you'll come to find out, I believe that maintaining a healthy metabolic rate and letting go of stress are two of the most important things that form the foundation of health. My experience is that restriction tends to worsen metabolic health and increase stress.

Therefore, unlike many other herbal books, in this book you won't find me telling you that sugar is bad or that fats are bad or any of the other nonsense that passes for health information these days. Rather, you'll hopefully understand that I advocate for listening to your body to determine your needs.

I learned to listen to my body the hard way. I became desperately sick. I had been trying very hard to get well, but nothing was helping. As a long-time believer in plant medicine, I had been using herbs to try to help myself, but eventually I became too weak for even the herbs to help me.

It was then that I discovered the tremendous importance of metabolism and hormonal health. It is my belief that when metabolic rate is sufficiently impaired, it becomes virtually impossible for even the strongest herbs to help with most symptoms. Because of my own experience, I first want to share with you some simple steps you can take to improve metabolic health.

Hormonal health usually follows on the heels of metabolic health. This is not always the case. However, because hormonal health depends so strongly on metabolic health, I believe that focusing on metabolic health first and foremost is the most important thing. Then, when metabolic rate is normalized, if hormonal imbalances still seem to be present, it is possible to further address this with some other suggestions.

Herbs can then help tremendously with a great many conditions. I have long believed in the power of herbal medicine, but it wasn't until after I recovered from being so sick that I finally discovered how to really listen to and respect that medicine.

I have learned herbalism through relationships with the plants themselves; therefore, I can really only share with you honest, living knowledge of the herbs that I know. Of the herbs that I know, I choose to share with you only those that I not only personally benefit from, but that have also been the subject of human studies demonstrating that they are effective for other humans as well.

When I say that I have learned through relationships with the plants themselves, that doesn't mean that I hear voices from the plants (not that I dismiss that as a possibility, but it's not my experience). Rather, I have learned to listen to the language of the plants as they communicate with me. Often times, that simply takes the form of ingesting a plant and finding out what it feels like. It's not a difficult thing to do that is reserved for some strange folk. Any of us can do it if we want to.

Some of the experiences have been wonderful. Some have been horrific. Most have been very mild. Up until I got very sick, I used to take a reckless approach. I would consume large amounts of strong herbs. In addition to herbs like chamomile, dandelion, and nettle that are relatively subtle in their action, I would also eat large amounts of herbs such as trichocereus peruvianus, amanita muscaria, and calamus. I used to believe that more is better and stronger is better. I used to believe that I had to have some sort of massive felt experience after consuming an herb in order to benefit.

Yet what I learned after far too many horrific bouts of nausea and terror is that this heroic approach to herbalism isn't for me. I don't believe there is much benefit in it other than finally discovering how to be grateful for every moment. After eight hours of fearing for annihilation, followed by a few hours of vomiting and diarrhea, it becomes easier to appreciate the wonder, joy, and beauty of just being alive.

After being very, very sick and near death, barely able to move for several years following a bacterial infection called Lyme disease, I came to appreciate the value of combining metabolic health with hormonal health with gentle, nourishing herbs to bring about a bodily balance that makes it easier to enjoy the amazing gift of life.

In this book, I hope to share with you the insights that have helped me to discover health after years of sickness. And I hope to share with you some simple ways to use gentle, nourishing herbs to address some common men's concerns.

I do not intend for this to be a definitive men's herbal. Rather, it is meant to be a simplification of herbs for men based on my own experiences. Are there other herbs and other valid ideas out there? Sure. My belief, however, is that much of that is unnecessary. A lot of the herbs that are marketed to men are marketed to make money, not necessarily to really help. So my hope is that what I share with you in this book will not only benefit your health, but also benefit your wallet by keeping you safe from predatory marketing techniques.

There are three parts to this book. In the first part, I share with you my findings and experiences on a variety of conditions and subjects. Initially, I share with you my findings in regard to metabolic health. Then, you'll find herbal advice on dealing with subjects such as urinary and prostate conditions, thyroid function, hair loss, stress, and insulin sensitivity.

In the second part of the book, I share with you how to use herbal medicine, as well as profiles of some of my favorite herbs.

Lastly, I share with you a collection of resources that you may find helpful.

I share with you honest information that I have discovered through my own experience and "verified" through research. However, just because I say so (or just because anyone else says so) doesn't make it true or true for you. The herbs and suggestions that I share with you in this book are all generally quite safe. However, that doesn't mean that some people may not find adverse reactions to some of the herbs or suggestions. So always listen to your body, listen to your intuition, and explore the suggestions with prudence and intelligence. No heroics are necessary.

Some Definitions

To begin with, let's make sure that we're all on the same page with some basic definitions before we get to the rest of the material in the book.

It is possible to view the actions of herbs in a variety of ways. I believe that each way of seeing has its own merits. And, when all views are considered, we have a more holistic and inclusive way to perceive ourselves and our relationships to others, including plants.

So let it be known that I fully believe that there are ways in which plants communicate with us that cannot be captured through the reductionist approach. And yet, these ways of communicating are best captured experientially with an open mind and an open heart or through poetry and song.

The reductionist approach is to attempt to view something through the sum of its parts. The reductionist view of herbs and their actions within the human organism seeks to view both herbs and humans as chemicals and the reactions between those chemicals. This is not the whole of what is happening, but it can be very useful. And, frankly, most of what you'll find in this book examines conditions and herbs in a rather reductionist approach.

From a reductionist standpoint, the human body has lots of systems and parts, and there are some very important substances that the body uses to communicate between systems and parts. Two types of substances of this sort that we'll look at in this book are hormones and cytokines.

When we think of hormones, many of us first think of sex hormones, such as testosterone or estrogen. Yet there are many other important hormones in our bodies. Some of those hormones include thyroid hormones, stress hormones, and insulin. We'll learn more about all of these types of hormones throughout the book.

Cytokines are specialized proteins that are used for communication in the body, and they play a crucial role in immunity. All of the types of cytokines play an important role in immunity, though in many cases of chronic illnesses and discomforts of various sorts, what has happened is that anti-inflammatory cytokines have become suppressed, while inflammatory cytokines are over-expressed. In this book, we'll look at ways to reduce inflammation and regulate immunity to improve health.

We'll also be looking at the importance of metabolism in this book. Broadly, metabolism is the collection of processes by which your body produces and uses energy. When metabolism is properly regulated, everything runs smoothly. When metabolism is low or high, problems ensue. So we'll be looking at ways to regulate metabolic rate as well.

Hormonal Health

Hormonal health plays a huge role in overall health. For example, too little or too much of thyroid hormones can completely wreak havoc with nearly every system in the body, producing problems with energy, anxiety, cognition, digestion, and more. When sex hormones are out of whack, this can produce many problems as well, including some types of cancer, hair loss, apathy, depression, and more. So hormonal health is a really big deal, and most herbal books fail to really examine its importance and the role that herbs can play in either exacerbating or improving hormonal health.

In this book, we'll look fairly extensively at regulating thyroid hormones and sex hormones. We'll also explore, briefly, insulin, which is a hormone that gets a lot of (negative) attention.

Inflammation

We've all experienced inflammation of various sorts, including sprains, fractures, scrapes, cuts, bruises, and so forth.

What few of us realize is that inflammation, despite being painful and unpleasant, is actually an important part of the healing process. Inflammation is managed by cytokines. When things are working properly, the correct balance of inflammatory and anti-inflammatory cytokines produce just the right amount of inflammation at just the right time in order to produce the necessary healing effects.

The trouble is when we are experiencing chronic inflammation. This can look like carpal tunnel syndrome, chronic headaches, arthritis, myalgia, and other chronic aches and pains. Perhaps surprisingly, it can also look like a lot of other things that we don't necessarily normally associate with inflammation - things such as insulin resistance, heart troubles, anxiety, cognitive impairment, and even mood instability. I am not suggesting that these problems are always only caused by inflammation. However, inflammation can and does play a significant role in many cases of chronic illness, disease, and discomfort.

Because of this, understanding inflammation and how to reduce chronic inflammation can be important in healing from all kinds of chronic ailments.

Immunity

The immune system, as we conceive of it, is the natural defense system of the body. This is how your body protects itself from a variety of concerns that could compromise health. This system includes everything from surface barriers (i.e. skin) to mechanical and chemical barriers (i.e. tears and mucous) to cellular barriers (i.e. white blood cells) to inflammatory processes and so on. There are many layers of immunity. It also includes the lymphatic system, which can function as the waste removal system - disinfected pathogens or other material that the immune system has deemed inappropriate to keep are ushered out through this system.

There are plenty of things that could theoretically compromise the immune system in one way or another. Fundamentally, if you are healthy overall, then minor problems tend to self-correct. For example, a surface wound (i.e. a cut in the skin) is a theoretical compromise to the immune system.

However, most of the time this self-corrects. Likewise, a temporary dryness of the mucous membranes can, theoretically, compromise the immune system, but in a healthy individual this will self-correct.

The main problem that we'll look at in this book is when cytokine expression becomes dysregulated. The result of this is, most often, a chronic inflammatory response (which breaks down tissue) and/or an elevated allergic response. Both of these may be caused by over-expression of some cytokines and possibly the suppression of others.

In the big picture, the best strategy for improving immunity is to modulate cytokine expression. In this book, we'll look at how herbs can support that. It's worth noting also that low metabolic rate, hormonal imbalance, and stress can all strongly influence immunity negatively. So balancing and regulating immunity in the long-term requires restoring balance across the board.

Metabolism

Metabolism refers to the processes by which your body produces energy and maintains all the functions of the body. Just as an engine must be throttled just right to maintain correct function, so too must the metabolism be tuned just right. If the metabolism is too high or too low, then everything will be out of whack, including immunity, hormonal health, stress response, and just about everything else.

Metabolism adapts to various circumstances. For example, during the initial stages of most infections, metabolism will increase. Yet chronic illness can lower metabolism. Likewise, stress can increase metabolism initially, yet sustained, chronic stress lowers metabolism.

Of all the factors that affect metabolism, however, the one that seems to have the most influence is how much dietary energy one is taking in. Those who chronically undereat typically have lowered metabolic rates. On the other hand, those who eat large amounts on a regular basis may have increased metabolic rates. For example, there are many athletes who regularly consume as much as 10,000 calories every day while training. Although these athletes do use a lot of that energy due to increased activity, much of the energy gets used as a result of an increased metabolic rate.

In my own experience, metabolism (specifically the metabolic rate) plays a huge role in overall health. I ended up increasingly sick over the course of many years until I was nearly dead. I had tried many approaches to solve my health problems, and yet nothing worked until I understood the importance of metabolic rate. For this reason, I view that metabolism is fundamental to most every health issue we can experience. Metabolism can greatly influence hormonal balance, digestion, emotional health, and more. And while herbs can offer powerful medicine to help with many conditions, I find that if metabolic rate is problematic, then there is often very little that anything, including some very powerful herbs, can do. This is why I propose to you that understanding metabolic health is an essential foundation for anything else that follows in this book.

When everything is working well, the metabolic rate is such that all the functions of the body such as digestion, heart rate, respiration, hormone production, and so forth are working smoothly. And the metabolism may increase or decrease its rate within a small range in order to meet changing needs. For example, metabolic rate tends to increase during early stages of infection or while running up a hill, and it tends to decrease naturally when sleeping. Yet this is a relatively small range of change and only for a short time.

Metabolic rate can rise or fall chronically (i.e. the basal metabolic rate may change), and this tends to lead to many problems. Again, if you consider the throttle for an engine, then you can see how if the throttle is stuck in a closed or wide open position, then this may lead to lots of problems with the engine.

Although it is possible to have a hypermetabolic state (chronically high metabolic rate), it is more common that metabolic rate is too low, which is called a hypometabolic state. Either case is problematic.

Hypermetabolism may be brought on by various circumstances, though some of the most common are hyperthyroid conditions. Hypermetabolism is also seen as a temporary condition during refeeding following starvation, though in this case, once the person eats enough consistently enough, the metabolic rate will return to a balanced and healthy state.

Hypometabolism too has many potential causes. Hypometabolism can be brought about by low thyroid function, starvation, chronic infection, and many other factors.

As best I can tell, hypermetabolism is very rare in comparison to rates of hypometabolism. And because some of the main causes of hypermetabolism are thyroid disorders, I will refer you to the discussion of thyroid health for insights on how to address hypermetabolism.

Hypometabolism, on the other hand, can result in the following symptoms:

- insomnia or disturbed sleep (often waking in the early morning with symptoms of high cortisol and/or adrenaline)
- depression
- anxiety
- food sensitivities or intolerances
- leaky gut
- irritable bowel
- edema or fluid retention
- intolerance to cold (and sometimes heat)
- cold hands and feet
- low or non-existent sex drive
- memory and/or cognitive problems
- dry skin, possibly rashes
- muscle and joint pain

- falling hair
- weight gain or weight loss (weight gain is more typical, but weight loss can result, particularly in chronic hypometabolic cases when a person has difficulty consuming enough food)
- frequent urination - particularly at night
- fatigue

One of the simplest ways I have found to measure metabolic rate is to record basal body temperature and resting pulse every morning before getting out of bed for a week. Record one or two body temperature readings throughout the day each of those days as well. Low temperature or low pulse typically indicate low metabolic rate. Experts vary on what they consider to be low, however, a basal temperature (which must be read without having slept with electric blankets or on a waterbed or anything else that would artificially elevate temperature) of less than 97.8 degrees Fahrenheit is generally considered to be low, while temperatures during the day that are under 98.6 degrees Fahrenheit may be considered low. A resting pulse under 65 beats per minute is considered low.

If you have a low metabolic rate and any of the symptoms from the preceding list, then you may see improvements in symptoms if you can increase metabolic rate.

The next task is to try and determine what the possible cause of low metabolic rate may be. At this point it becomes interesting, because some of the very things that can cause low metabolic rate can also be symptoms of low metabolic rate. For example, infection can cause low metabolic rate and, at the same time, low metabolic rate can lower immunity and make one more susceptible to chronic infection. Similarly, low thyroid function can cause hypometabolism, yet hypometabolism can also cause low thyroid function.

What I find to be a very reasonable approach is to try and address metabolism through the most direct means possible first, before trying to solve other problems that you suspect may be at cause. And the most direct way that I know of to address metabolism is with food.

There are two key ways to suppress metabolism with food. One is not to eat enough. The other is to eat large amounts of metabolism-suppressing foods and/or restrict foods that nourish the metabolism. Likewise, it is often possible to improve metabolic function by eating enough and by eating foods that nourish metabolism while reducing foods that suppress metabolism.

I discovered some studies that monitored what healthy, weight-stable humans eat (versus what they report eating), and the results were surprising. People typically under report how much they eat, sometimes by as much as 58%. When we extrapolate the results, here are the implications: men under the age of 25 actually eat 3500 calories or more a day. Men age 25 and over actually eat 3000 calories a day or more. And the more active men are, the more they need to eat.

When I learned that, I realized that my suppressed metabolic rate could have been from eating too little. So I committed to an experiment of eating at least 3000 calories every day, and within days I started to feel much better. As the months went by, I continued to feel better.

It is helpful to eat foods that nourish metabolic health. Many of us have fallen into the trap of trying to eat healthfully, which usually means restricting in one way or another. Some of us restrict macronutrients by restricting fat or carbohydrates, and usually all macronutrients are necessary to support a healthy metabolism. So if you are restricting macronutrients and experiencing hypometabolic conditions, then you may want to consider the impact that diet can have. Proteins, saturated fats, cholesterol, starch, sugar, and salt all seem to be necessary for a healthy metabolism in the long run.

Foods that seem to harm metabolic rate include polyunsaturated fats (such as corn or canola oil), soy, excessive bran, and excessive brassicas (such as broccoli or kale)

I personally feel that much of what pretends to be health information turns out to be more harmful than helpful. We're led to believe that we should be eating lots of soy, flax, canola oil, and green smoothies for optimal health, but when we eat based on ideologies like that, I see that more often than not it causes problems in the long run.

My goal in this book is not to write extensively about nutrition, and so I will not attempt to write a long explanation of how much of the science behind most of the health claims for so-called "health" food is unfounded and discredited. You can find that elsewhere. My hope with this section on metabolic health is simply to give you some information that you can use to determine if metabolic rate may be a problem for you. And if that seems likely, then how you can at least consider some simple dietary changes to improve metabolic rate. Basically, you can see it as an experiment that you can explore for a few weeks to see what sort of changes you notice, if any, by making some dietary changes. The dietary changes that I recommend are to let up on the restrictions, include all macronutrients, eat according to desire rather than ideology, enjoy metabolism-nourishing foods, and ease up on the foods that suppress metabolism. For most people, this is rather enjoyable. After all, most of us would rather eat cheesy potatoes fried in butter rather than a kale and tofu smoothie.

Thyroid

Although you're not likely to hear nearly as much about the thyroid as you are, say, the heart or the liver or the prostate, you may be surprised to discover the important influence that this small gland exerts over your entire body and mind. It determines how the body uses energy and hormones. It is the master regulator. When the thyroid is functioning well, it is easier for the rest of the body to function well - like an engine can function well when the throttle is properly set. But when the thyroid is not functioning optimally - either overactive or underactive - this sets the stage for all kinds of problems affecting everything from energy levels to digestion to mood to sleep and more.

Even by conservative estimates, hypothyroidism (underactive thyroid) affects nearly five times as many people as hyperthyroidism (overactive thyroid). And there are some who believe that the numbers for hypothyroidism are actually much higher due to the conservative medical tests for low thyroid function - namely, insufficient thyroid hormones detected in the blood.

However, it is challenging to really determine if the thyroid is where the difficulty lies in most cases. Thyroid hormone tests don't always give satisfactory insights into why someone may be experiencing symptoms of low thyroid. And while some people claim that temperature and resting pulse can be used to diagnose thyroid health, it seems to me that these diagnostics measure metabolism, not thyroid. While there is often a close link between thyroid and metabolism, I don't believe that it is useful to conflate the two.

Therefore, I suggest that in the absence of either goiter (swelling of the thyroid, which is located in front of the throat) or hormone tests that show high or low thyroid hormones, it may be most profitable to consider metabolic health rather than thyroid health first and foremost. What follows is for your consideration if you have reason to believe that you may be experiencing thyroid dysfunction independent of metabolism.

Hypothyroidism

There are various causes of hypothyroidism. Reportedly, the most common cause of hypothyroidism in the United States is Hashimoto's disease. Other causes include iodine deficiency, congenital disease (born with an incomplete or malfunctioning thyroid), radiation, thyroid removal, medication, some other glandular diseases, and some infections.

Hashimoto's Disease

The advice from professionals and laypeople alike is far from a consensus when it comes to treating Hashimoto's disease. While most recommend against any supplemental iodine, such as might be found in sea vegetables like kelp or bladderwrack, there are a few who claim that iodine deficiency may actually be the cause of Hashimoto's. Anecdotally, many people with Hashimoto's disease find that dietary iodine makes their symptoms worse. So if you have been diagnosed with Hashimoto's disease, then I strongly caution against supplemental iodine without good reason.

The rest of the recommendations that I offer you in the following sections should be useful and applicable regardless of whether the cause of your hypothyroid condition is an autoimmune condition or not. You should be able to proceed with the other recommendations (non-iodine-containing) without concern. In other words, simply do not include sea vegetables in your diet if you have Hashimoto's disease and you have reason to suspect that additional iodine may contribute to worsening symptoms.

I will add that while medical professionals most commonly state that they honestly do not know what causes Hashimoto's disease, some professionals suggest that various infections may play an important role in causing or maintaining Hashimoto's. For example, the bacteria Yersinia enterocolitica has been implicated in some cases of Hashimoto's, while parvovirus B19 may be implicated in other cases. And, of course, there may be other organisms that could be causing the condition.

If this is true, then there are some herbs that may address the underlying infection. Which herbs will work will depend on the infecting organism. In the case of Yersinia enterocolitica, juniper and usnea could be very effective, though if the infection is systemic, then systemic antibacterial herbs may be more suitable (see antibacterial herbs section). For parovirus B19, I am not familiar with any studies that may shed light on what herbs could be helpful, though I suspect that systemic antibacterial herbs may help.

Also, in the case of Hashimoto's disease, a chronic inflammatory response is typically a cause of many of the problems. So reducing that chronic inflammatory response with the correct herbs may be very useful. Although I cannot find any studies specifically indicating that specific herbs reduce symptoms or causes of Hashimoto's disease (the research into the disease doesn't tend to go in that direction), I do find research indicating which inflammatory cytokines are elevated in the disease. It is reasonable to believe that reducing this inflammation safely will produce positive outcomes.

In fact, there is some anecdotal evidence (self-reporting from those with Hashimoto's disease) that anti-inflammatory herbs of the right sort can reduce symptoms or even, apparently, reverse the condition in some cases. Turmeric seems to be the best candidate, in my opinion. The reason that I like turmeric in this case is that it shows no thyroid suppressing activity and is strongly inhibitive of the specific inflammatory response in Hashimoto's disease. I recommend starting with 1/8 teaspoon of the dried turmeric powder 3 times a day and increase to 1/2 teaspoon 3 times a day, if you can tolerate it well and you see benefits.

I have read some reports of people using Japanese knotweed (or resveratrol extracted from Japanese knotweed) in combination with turmeric to address the inflammation in Hashimoto's disease. This may work for some people. I do like Japanese knotweed quite a lot, and I believe it is a powerful herb. However, I have reservations suggesting Japanese knotweed generally for this specific purpose because several compounds isolated from the herb (resveratrol and trans-resveratrol, which are thought to be the therapeutic compounds for reducing inflammation) also have thyroid suppressing activity.

So my advice is to begin with turmeric alone to reduce inflammation in cases of Hashimoto's disease.

Iodine Deficiency

As you likely know, iodine is an important mineral for thyroid health. In fact, the thyroid requires iodine in order to create thyroid hormones. So obviously, insufficient iodine can cause hypothyroidism. In fact, this is the reason we are told that table salt manufacturers often add iodine to the product: to help prevent iodine deficiency.

Medical establishment organizations, such as the National Institutes of Health, make vague claims such as that "iodine deficiency in North America is rare" or "iodine deficiency is uncommon." However, I have yet to see any actual data to back up these claims.

On the other hand, a minority of physicians claim that when they actually test patients, they find that as many as 96% are deficient in iodine.

With such a huge discrepancy, it's hard to sort out truth from fiction here. It is also difficult to figure out what is the most accurate way to test for iodine deficiency. What does seem clear is that the so-called "patch test," involving "painting" a patch of skin with iodine and observing the length of time it takes to disappear, is not a reliable or accurate test. And, furthermore, the standard urine test for iodine is suspect and doesn't likely yield reliable results.

This leaves two other types of tests - blood tests or the iodine load test. My research suggests that blood tests for iodine are not standard, so if you are having blood work done and you want the lab to test for iodine, then you need to make that request. The iodine load test is a urine test that uses a special protocol whereby the patient ingests substantial supplemental iodine during a 24-hour period prior to the test. You can learn more about how to do a load test by searching on the internet for "iodine load test."

What is notable is that since the addition of iodine to table salt, the overall numbers for hypothyroidism have continued to increase bit by bit, according to the statistics I have come across. While it may be purely coincidental, during this same time period, we can see that our environmental exposure to other halogens (namely fluoride, chlorine, and bromine) that compete for space in the body with iodine has continued to increase. Many municipalities add fluoride and chlorine to water supplies, and bromine is found in many flour products (such as bread), as well as in flame retardants added to furniture, bedding, and clothing.

One theory as to the increased incidences of hypothyroidism suggests that with all the exposure to competing halogens, modern humans are overloaded with fluoride, chlorine, and bromine and thus do not absorb dietary iodine. Whether or not this explains everything, it certain does seem prudent to take reasonable steps to reduce your exposure to competing halogens. If possible, drink and bathe in non-fluoridated, non-chlorinated water. Otherwise, at least run your drinking water through a carbon filter to remove much of the chlorine. (Any carbon filter should do a decent job of removing chlorine. Filters to remove fluoride, on the other hand, are pricier than simple carbon filters, and frankly, you pretty much have to take the manufacturer's word that they work as advertised since there aren't any inexpensive fluoride testers on the market for you to test the results yourself.) You can reduce your bromine exposure by choosing unbromated flour and products and choosing either untreated furniture or used furniture, which has already off-gassed much of the flame retardants.

Another obstacle to iodine uptake are substances called goitrogens that appear in a variety of common foods. Goitrogens may block iodine absorption in the thyroid even in the presence of large amounts of dietary iodine, so it is generally a good idea to minimize dietary goitrogens if you have thyroid problems. Some of the foods with the most significant quantities of goitrogens are brassicas (broccoli, cabbage, kale, turnips, mustard, canola, etc.), soy, cassava/tapioca, millet, sweet potatoes, strawberries, peaches, and pears. Although you needn't avoid these foods entirely, it may be a good idea to minimize them in your diet temporarily while you are having problems with thyroid health.

There are many claims on the internet that goitrogens are eliminated or deactivated by cooking and fermentation. However, in my research, neither of these claims are true. As best I can tell, cooking does not deactivate goitrogens. If you cook foods in water and discard the water, then you can, perhaps, reduce the goitrogen content in the food because you will discard the goitrogens that leach into the water. And from my research, fermentation (as in kimchi and sauerkraut) actually increases goitrogen content.

Of course, if you reduce your exposure to competing halogens and you reduce your consumption of goitrogens but you are deficient in iodine, then you will continue to have thyroid problems. Now, unfortunately, there seems to be a great deal of misinformation as well as political agendas that make it difficult for most of us to sort out the truth when it comes to iodine. There are some physicians who argue that iodine deficiency is a widespread, silent epidemic and that supplementing with massive amounts of iodine (50 mg or even as much as 200 mg per day) is perfectly safe and essential for many people. On the other hand, there is a more conservative majority that suggests that we need very little iodine (150 mcg per day) and that excessive iodine is harmful. Sadly, it's extremely difficult to sort out the facts from the fiction when it comes to supplemental iodine. My own personal belief based upon much study of this subject is that our actual iodine needs are quite small, and extreme supplementation is likely more harmful than helpful in most cases. That doesn't mean that it may not help in some cases, of course. But the one-size-fits-all approach of large doses of iodine proposed by some seems reckless to me.

What does seem true is that if you have a clear iodine deficiency and you do not have an autoimmune disorder affecting your thyroid, then supplementing with iodine can be an important step in restoring health. Otherwise, however, increasing your intake of iodine may cause you more problems.

Here it gets confusing, because a minority of physicians suggest that some of the problems that people experience when increasing iodine intake are actually the result of other halogens from the body getting displaced by the iodine (which would be potentially positive) and thus causing unpleasant symptoms in the short term until they are properly metabolized and excreted. It is difficult to know what is really going on, but what does seem clear is that some people respond poorly to increasing intake of iodine. Typically, the people who respond poorly are not clearly iodine deficient. So, if you want to play it safe, you can get an iodine urine test to determine if you are deficient.

For those who are wishing to supplement with iodine, then the best herbal options are herbs from the ocean as most of these herbs have high levels of iodine. Kelp and bladderwrack are among the most popular herbs for this purpose.

Other herbs that contain significant levels of iodine include white oak bark and black walnut hulls. Black walnut hulls are traditionally used only short-term because of the potentially unwanted side effects when used long-term.

Heavy Metals

Heavy metals, such as mercury, arsenic, cadmium, aluminum, and lead, are thought to cause many health problems, including low thyroid function. While some alternative health practitioners take an alarmist stance in regard to the dangers of heavy metals, most medical professionals take a much more conservative and dismissive stance. As with most things, the truth may be somewhere in between but it's difficult to know what the truth is with all the politics.

Since many of us are exposed to heavy metals in non-trivial amounts through various means, if you suspect that you have low thyroid function, then it may be prudent to use some herbs for the purpose of assisting your body in excreting excess heavy metals in a natural and balanced way.

Unlike the aggressive and potentially depleting and unbalancing chemical chelating agents such as DMSA and EDTA, the recommendations that I offer you are natural and should be very gentle and balanced. These herbs should help create and maintain a positive mineral balance in your body.

Silica is an important element for heavy metal detoxification. Many herbalists recommend horsetail as a silica-rich herb. In fact, when horsetail is planted in soil that contains high levels of heavy metals, it can remove the heavy metals from the soil. Some people have even been known to burn horsetail and extract gold from the ash, so theoretically, horsetail may be a useful herb for detoxifying heavy metals. Personally, I have limited personal experience with the herb. I have not used it long-term, and I cannot attest to its safety long-term. I personally feel more comfortable with calcium bentonite clay suitable for internal use. Calcium bentonite clay is high in silica and other minerals, and I find it to be a very powerful supplement.

Garlic has a long history as a detoxifying herb, and recent studies show that garlic does, in fact, help to chelate various heavy metals. While some like to claim that garlic must be eaten raw or in special extract form to gain the benefits, research suggests that any form of garlic has benefits. So cooking with garlic is likely to be both beneficial and more palatable than eating raw cloves. In fact, much of the research suggests that the sulfur compounds found in garlic may be responsible for the benefits. If that is so, then onions and brassicas may also be helpful in a similar fashion. However, for low thyroid function, brassicas may be contraindicated since they contain compounds known as goitrogens that can suppress thyroid function.

Yarrow is an herb that contains the mineral selenium and is beneficial for male hormonal balance. Selenium is shown to help chelate mercury from the brain, so theoretically, including yarrow in your herbal regimen may help with chelating heavy metals while also helping to balance hormones.

Brown sea vegetables, such as kelp, contain substances called algal polysaccharides alginate that have demonstrated the ability to chelate heavy metals. Theoretically, adding kelp to your diet may support heavy metal chelation. Although there are cultures that traditionally have eaten sea vegetables on a daily basis, there is some debate about whether eating sea vegetables every day is advisable due to the iodine content. Personally, I doubt that reasonable amounts of sea vegetables are likely to be a problem for most people. However, if you have doubts, then listen to your body's needs, and be respectful. Also, we are led to believe that the oceans are now terribly polluted with industrial waste, which has raised the heavy metal levels in the ocean to dangerous levels. My suspicion is that the sea vegetables are mopping up the heavy metals, which likely increases the heavy metal concentrations in the vegetables. However, it is also likely that they have additional chelating capacity still, and therefore will still chelate heavy metals from those who eat them. I do not know whether this is true or not, however, so caveat emptor.

Citrus peels, such as orange peels or lemon peels, contain a substance called pectin that has been shown to chelate heavy metals and help to excrete them.

Ginger has demonstrated some effectiveness is chelating some heavy metals in mice, though I don't know of any human studies. So ginger may be helpful, though to what degree we don't really know. I wouldn't rely on ginger as a sole chelator, though in combination with others it may be quite effective.

Cilantro is an herb that has become quite popular for eliminating excess heavy metals. However, the studies have not backed the claims about the chelating power of the herb. In fact, some studies show that cilantro is no more effective than placebo. I happen to rather enjoy cilantro, and so I grow it and eat it. If you enjoy cilantro, then by all means eat it, however, I am skeptical of the expensive "chelating" supplements that include cilantro as the main ingredient. I recommend against trying to use cilantro for the purposes of chelating heavy metals.

Chlorella, which is a type of algae, is another substance that studies suggest may be effective in chelating heavy metals. However, this so-called "superfood" is hardly a traditional food since it requires industrial processes to break the cell walls and make it digestible to humans. We simply don't know what the long-term effects of consuming chlorella are for humans. Plus, it is a fairly expensive supplement, so I recommend skipping it.

Additional Herbs for Hypothyroidism

In addition to the herbs mentioned in the preceding sections, there are a few more herbs that stand out as having substantial potential to help with hypothyroid conditions.

Ashwagandha is an herb with a long history of use in the Ayurvedic tradition that has many potential uses, including the potential to modulate thyroid activity. There are several studies that show that ashwagandha can increase sluggish thyroid function.

Nettle leaf can also support thyroid health and may improve thyroid hormone conversion.

Milk thistle seed is also shown to be supportive of a slow thyroid. Furthermore, milk thistle seed is a powerful liver protectant.

Supporting liver health is important for hypothyroidism because 80% of thyroid hormone conversion takes place in the liver. So see the section on liver health for more information on supporting the liver. For Hashimoto's disease, turmeric is a natural because it can reduce inflammation and support the liver. Milk thistle seed is a natural because it may directly support the thyroid, and it protects the liver.

The aforementioned herbs in this section are gentle and should be safe for just about anyone. The herbs that follow are still relatively gentle and safe, and they are herbs that I personally use on a regular (though not every single day) basis. However, these herbs may exert a stronger effect in stimulating the thyroid than the previously mentioned herbs. Do not expect reasonable doses of these herbs to create hyperthyroid conditions. They shouldn't be that strong. I find them to be tonic herbs that are safe for regular use. Just be cautious if you have any history of hyperthyroidism, and start with low doses and increase slowly.

Guggul is another herb with a long tradition in Ayurveda. There is some evidence that suggests that guggul may be useful for hypothyroid conditions. Guggul is said to increase T4 to T3 conversion, which is very useful for those who have enough T4 but are T3 deficient. (T4 and T3 are thyroid hormones with T3 said to be the "active" form.)

Bacopa is another herb that can stimulate the thyroid. Bacopa reportedly increases T4 levels, but it may not increase T4 to T3 conversion.

Gotu kola is reported to increase thyroid function. I have yet to come across any studies that verify this, but anecdotal evidence is good that gotu kola is useful for supporting the thyroid in cases o hypothyroidism.

Finally, there is an herb called coleus forskohlii that may indirectly increase thyroid function. Coleus stimulates something called cAMP, which, in turn, increases thyroid output. So this may be helpful for improving low thyroid function, but I don't know of any long-term studies on the effects. I am currently working with the herb myself, and I have found it to be quite good with no unpleasant side effects. If you do decide to use coleus (it is being marketed rather aggressively at the moment as a weight loss herb, which really is ridiculous), then I strongly caution against using the standardized herb or the pure forskolin extract. Forskolin (the isolated compound said to be the "active ingredient" in the herb), has some drawbacks in high concentrations that are offset when it is buffered and in normal doses in the whole herb. So I encourage you to use only the whole herb or a full-spectrum extract.

Obviously, this list of herbs is not exhaustive. There are so many plants in the world that no list can ever be comprehensive. What I have included in these sections for hypothyroidism are the herbs that I am aware of and have used myself that demonstrate the ability to help with hypothyroid conditions.

In addition to the herbs I have listed for use in helping with hypothyroid conditions, I would also suggest that you should avoid any herbs that are known to suppress thyroid function, such as some of those listed in the next section, including bugleweed, lemon balm, and motherwort.

Also, those with hypothyroid conditions would likely do best to eat abundantly of most foods while keeping some of the notable thyroid-suppressing foods to a minimum. Foods that are thought to suppress thyroid function include goitrogenic foods (see list earlier in the book) and polyunsaturated fats (soy, corn, safflower, canola, and other similar vegetable oils).

Hyperthyroidism

Hyperthyroidism is a condition in which the thyroid is overactive, and, unlike hypothyroidism, the thyroid is creating too many hormones. The results can be not only unpleasant, but potentially life-threatening. Racing heart palpitations, particularly, can be a major problem.

Grave's disease is an autoimmune condition that is thought to be responsible for the majority of cases of hyperthyroidism. Like Hashimoto's disease, the causes of Grave's diseases are officially unknown, yet it is believed that bacterial or viral infections may be the cause in at least some cases. In fact, the same bacteria, Yersinia enterocolitica, is implicated in some cases of Grave's disease as it is in some cases of Hashimoto's disease.

If it is true that Yersinia enterocolitica is the cause of some cases of Grave's disease, then juniper and usnea may be helpful. It is also likely that in such a case the infection would be systemic, in which case systemic antibacterial herbs may be helpful.

Because Grave's disease is classified as an autoimmune condition that involves chronic inflammation, it may be very helpful to use an appropriate herb that effectively reduces the right sort of inflammation. This can slow or halt the autoimmune response. Turmeric is my best recommendation for treating the inflammation in Grave's disease. It should not affect thyroid hormone production directly, making it safe to use. However, it can powerfully reduce inflammation safely.

If turmeric does not provide sufficient anti-inflammatory relief, or if you are unable to tolerate turmeric for some reason, then Japanese knotweed may help. There is some evidence that Japanese knotweed may suppress thyroid function, which may make it helpful in reducing some symptoms of Grave's disease while also reducing inflammation. I have read some anecdotal reports of people using

Japanese knotweed (or resveratrol extract) in treating Grave's disease. However, I have not seen any studies on this subject, so caveat emptor.

Often times in cases of hyperthyroidism, medical professionals and herbalists alike recommend herbs that suppress thyroid function. At least in the short term, this may be helpful in reducing symptoms, but in the long run, it is unclear whether suppressing the thyroid is a useful approach.

Herbs that are traditionally used to suppress thyroid function include bugleweed, lemon balm, and motherwort. The first, bugleweed, is a bit of a mixed bag, and so I would suggest opting for the other herbs instead. In addition to suppressing thyroid function, the latter two both have sedative properties that may help with some of the symptoms of hyperthyroidism, such as insomnia, hyperactivity, and anxiety.

Most recommend avoiding extra iodine in cases of hyperthyroidism because this will exacerbate symptoms. Unless you have very good reason to do so, avoid large amounts of iodine, such as that found in sea vegetables.

Hyperthyroidism is linked with excess stress, so many professionals recommend learning stress-relief practices, which can greatly reduce symptoms. There are many great programs and practices for stress-relief, and that subject is far beyond the scope of this book to go into detail. However, under the Stress heading in the resources section of the book, I share with you what I believe to be some of the very best programs for learning skills to let go of stress.

Some herbs can also be helpful for reducing stress, and thus helping with hyperthyroidism in some cases. In addition to the herbs already mentioned (lemon balm and motherwort), there are other herbs that may be helpful to reduce stress without suppressing thyroid function. These herbs are discussed in the Stress section later in the book.

Sex Hormones

Sex hormones are a big deal. The delicate balance of androgens and estrogens can play an important role in everything from creative drive and motivation to hair loss and cancer.

The sex hormone that we most often hear about in connection with men is testosterone. However, testosterone is just one of a handful of hormones that play a vital role in men's health. These hormones are called androgens, and they include not only testosterone, but also DHEA, androsterone, androstenedione, androstenediol, and DHT. All of these androgens are important for male health.

Estrogens are the types of hormones that we normally associated with females. While it is true that women typically have a higher estrogen to androgen ratio than men, both men and women have both categories of hormones. Some amount of estrogens is important for male health. However, too much estrogen can cause problems for men, including even very serious health problems like cancer.

For men, the ideal is to maintain a healthy ratio of sex hormones in which there are more androgens than estrogens. Under ideal conditions, this is effortless. However, there are many factors that can throw off the balance of sex hormones.

Damage to gonadal tissue (such as castration) will inevitably upset hormone balance. Yet even less severe occurrences can result in imbalances in sex hormones. For example, chronic stress, malnourishment, undereating, infections, pesticide exposure, hormones in food, and lack of sleep are some of the common ways that sex hormone balance may be thrown off. In addition, some herbs may exert a pro-estrogenic or an anti-androgenic effect that can cause imbalances. And, if metabolic health or liver health is compromised, then proper hormone metabolism (i.e. excreting excess estrogen) may be impaired, resulting in hormonal imbalance.

Let's look at some of the things you can do to bring about better hormonal balance. We'll look at some simple lifestyle choices that you can do as well as herbal approaches.

In terms of lifestyle choices that can support hormonal balance, here are some of the things you must do:

Learning effective strategies for letting go of stress can work miracles on sex hormone balance. As I suggested earlier, this is a subject well beyond the scope of this book, and there are many good practices and programs to help with this. See the Resources section of the book for my recommendations.

Malnourishment and undereating are two sure-fire ways to hurt hormonal balance. If you wish to restore balance, then it is often essential that you eat enough and that you eat a variety of foods. It isn't necessary or even helpful to adhere to a "pure" and restrictive diet of only "healthy" foods. Rather, it seems that what is important is to eat enough of all macronutrients (protein, fat, and carbohydrates) to fuel a healthy metabolism, and then to eat sufficient amounts of nutrient-dense foods. Nutrient-dense foods needn't make up all of your diet. Yet including butter, bone broth, whole milk, egg yolks, and organ meats to a diet that is diverse and includes enough calories can help provide both the energy and the nutrients the body needs to produce sex hormones. Sex hormones require adequate cholesterol, saturated fat, and protein.

Reduce your exposure to chemical pesticides (which are known endocrine disruptors) by choosing not to use them yourself and by choosing foods that are produced without them. You can also reduce your exposure to hormones and drugs that can upset hormone balance in your food by choosing meat and dairy that come from animals that were raised without drugs.

Also, making enough time to get adequate daily sleep is essential for hormonal balance. Androgen levels plummet without enough sleep. For most people, this means getting at least 8 hours of sleep every night.

For more information about herbs for stress, infection, and supporting restful sleep, see the relevant sections later in this book.

One other non-herbal approach to increasing androgens is exercise. However, it must be the right sort of exercise. Steady-state cardio (long distance running, cycling, etc.) actually causes hormonal havoc, and so it is a terrible idea for improving hormone balance. Compound (meaning that they work multiple muscle groups) resistance exercises (weight lifting) increase androgen levels. Lower body exercises, such as squats, increase androgen levels more than upper body exercises. The key to success in this endeavor is that the exercises must be short in duration (i.e. few repetitions), involve heavy weights, and allow for lots of rest and nutrition.

Some herbs are known to reduce androgens and/or increase estrogens. The two that most of the studies I have come across seem to confirm to be among the worst offenders are licorice and hops. For any man concerned about imbalances in sex hormones, you may be well advised to use licorice and hops sparingly, if at all. Hops, as we all know, are a common ingredient in most commercial beers.

I had previously reported that black cohosh also increased estrogens, but I have subsequently come across several studies that report that, in fact, despite widely held beliefs, black cohosh neither contains estrogens nor increases estrogens in the body.

Other herbs that may be problematic include alfalfa, clover, soy, and flax. All of these are known to contain phytoestrogens. Some suggest that these estrogen-like substances act as weak estrogens in the human body, thereby actually reducing the effects of estrogens. Yet there is also evidence that suggests that these herbs may problematic, so I suggest using them only if you have a very good reason.

On the other hand, there are herbs that are said to improve androgen to estrogen ratios in men. Some of these herbs are exotics that are marketed in such a way as to prey on men's insecurities or to suggest rather fantastical results. Most of these herbs are questionable in my view. Here are a few of the herbs commonly marketed to "increase testosterone":

Bulbine natalensis is an herb from South Africa that is receiving a lot of attention at present in bodybuilding circles. While the studies do demonstrate that the herb may increase androgen levels in rats, this doesn't necessarily translate to humans. Furthermore, there is some evidence that the herb may be harmful to the liver and kidneys, so

I feel that not enough is yet known about this herb to recommend it.

Eurycoma longifolia, also known as tongkat ali and longjack, is an herb from southeast Asia that reportedly does increase androgens in rats. However, whether it has the same effect in humans is unknown. I have also read reports that claim that much of the herb is contaminated with high levels of mercury, so I do not recommend this herb at this time.

Tribulus terrestris is a traditional herb that has recently received a lot of attention with claims that it boosts testosterone production. However, the studies do not demonstrate that this is so in humans. I do believe that tribulus is a safe and beneficial herb, as you will read later in the book. However, I do not believe that the claims that tribulus increases androgen production are substantiated, and mostly I believe the claims are just used to market cheap products to men.

Fenugreek is a leguminous seed that is used both for culinary and medicinal purposes. It is a beautiful plant that I have grown, and I do believe that it is a good herb for some purposes. However, testosterone production doesn't seem to be one of those uses. The only human study that I know of showed no increase in androgens as a result of the herb, though the researchers did find that the herb increased libido and sperm count.

Muira Puama is an Amazonian herb that has a long history of use among traditional people. The herb may have many benefits, but I cannot find any evidence that the herb does actually have a positive influence on sex hormone balance, so I cannot recommend it for this purpose.

Epimedium, also known as horny goat weed, is an herb with a long history of use in Chinese herbalism. While the herb does demonstrate the ability to increase libido and erectile strength, I do not know of any evidence that it has a positive influence on sex hormone balance. In fact, I have seen some studies that actually implicate this herb in increasing estrogen! And so, once again, I cannot recommend this herb for the purpose of balancing sex hormones.

Mucuna Pruriens, also known as cow vetch and velvet bean, among other names, is an herb that is most commonly used to treat Parkinson's disease. However, the herb has a reputation for being useful for everything from psychedelic experiences to lucid dreaming to increasing testosterone. Interestingly, there may be some evidence to support the claim that the herb can increase androgens. I know of several studies that show that the herb can increase androgen levels in rats. Of course, this doesn't mean that it will necessarily have the same effect in humans. However, there is at least one study that tested androgen levels in human males who were taking an herbal supplement that included mucuna pruriens. The trouble with the study is that it does not show definitively that the effects were the result of mucuna pruriens since there were two other herbs included in the supplement, but mucuna pruriens is the most likely candidate for the effects. Mucuna pruriens is an herb with a long history of safe use, and so it may be a good candidate for increasing androgens. Of all the herbs so far, this is the one that looks most promising. My personal opinion is that mucuna may be best suited for people with Parkinson's or some other obvious need, such as extremely low androgen levels, and it may be best avoided by otherwise healthy people who are merely seeking to improve androgen levels slightly. The reason is that as far as I can tell, the herb may possibly only work for this purpose (as well as any hormonal modulation, including adjusting dopamine for Parkinson's disease) when raw. However, the raw herb also contains some toxic substances, such as trypsin inhibitors. It tastes horrible, in my opinion (it is, after all, a raw bean), and it can make some people nauseous. Also, since it really can have a powerful effect on hormones of all sorts, I would only use it if I really had a strong need.

Pine is said to have large amounts of phytoandrogens, which are most concentrated in the pollen. For this reason, there are now many who are jumping on the bandwagon, claiming that pine pollen can increase androgens in human males. Herbalist

Stephen Buhner has written two books extolling the benefits of pine pollen for men, and he claims that there are human studies published in Chinese (though not yet translated into English) that bear out the claim that pine pollen can increase androgens in human males. He also gives anecdotal evidence that apparently female fish downstream from pine pulp mills become male due to the phytoandrogen content of the pulp released into the water.

And so, pine pollen does seem promising. However, at this time I cannot personally recommend it based on the lack of research in English that I can read and verify. While pine has a long history of use in Chinese herbalism, and surely it has many benefits, I cannot verify that it truly does have a favorable influence on sex hormone health in human males.

With all that said, pine is one of the most abundant trees across North America, which is where I live and where most of the readers of this book likely live. I have lived all over North America, and everywhere that I have lived - even here in the high desert of New Mexico - there are pines. As such, there is a great opportunity for many of us to collect pine pollen for ourselves. Since it is unlikely to do any harm to most of us, then pine pollen may be a wonderful herb that we can wild harvest ourselves. There is no financial cost to this (unlike the pricey tinctures available on the internet), and it is a fantastic opportunity for us to connect with the plants themselves. This offers us an opportunity to cultivate a relationship with the plants and learn of their nature, such as when, where, and how to collect the pollen.

Finally, there are some herbs that may help with clearing excess estrogen from the body. Since the liver is one of the primary sites where estrogen is metabolized, most of these herbs are herbs that improve liver function. See the Liver section later in the book for more insights into how to improve liver function.

Many claims are made that passionflower can reduce estrogen levels in the body due to the presence of a substance called chrysin. While the theory may be a good one, the only studies that I have found suggest that, in reality, passionflower has no effect on estrogen levels.

Likewise, there are many claims that chamomile can reduce estrogen levels in the body. However, I know of no studies that demonstrate that chamomile has this effect. In fact, chamomile also contains estrogenic compounds in addition to the substance that supposedly removes estrogen from the body. So what is most likely is that the substances in chamomile produce a balanced hormonal effect.

The herb self-heal (prunella vulgaris) has demonstrated the ability to reduce estrogen levels in rats. This does not translate to efficacy in humans, of course. However, since self-heal grows abundantly in the wild in many places, I mention it because it may be a good candidate for wild harvesting. And since it is an herb with a long tradition as a health-giving plant without any major side-effects, I would suggest that no harm is likely to come to you by wild harvesting self-heal from natural areas (no pesticides or other toxins) and eating it. If self-heal does have similar effects in humans as those seen in rats, then it may help balance estrogen levels. One word of caution, however: self-heal may suppress thyroid function, and therefore, it may be contraindicated in cases of hypothyroidism.

By the way, most foods and herbs have some effect on sex hormones. When you search the internet or consult various studies, you may find that some people will claim that dandelion or milk thistle or turmeric or eleuthero or nettle or any number of other herbs may increase or decrease androgens or estrogens. While this may be true (or may not be true), what I find is that with few notable exceptions, the majority of herbs have a rather neutral effect. For example, while milk thistle seed may increase estrogen, it also improves liver function, which increases estrogen clearance. So overall, I suspect that the effect is neutral or perhaps balancing (i.e. if there are excessive estrogens, then this may balance that by clearing more estrogen from the body). I don't absolutely know any of that to be true, though I suspect that it is.

In conclusion, it seems to me that the best way to use herbs to support sex hormone balance is to nourish the body using tonic herbs such as those that are discussed throughout the rest of the book. Most of the herbs that are touted as increasing androgens are unproven, and some are potentially dangerous. Herbs such as tribulus and fenugreek are not shown to increase androgens, though they may play a role in nourishing the body.

Overall, I recommend that the best strategies for improving sex hormone balance are sleeping, eating, letting go of stress, and nourishing the body with tonic herbs such as tribulus and ashwagandha. Weight-resistant compound exercise, especially emphasizing the lower body, also increases androgens.

Reducing Chronic Inflammation

When we think of inflammation, we normally think of pain, irritation, and even rashes (this includes things like sprains, breaks, fractures, bruises, arthritis, myalgias, and so forth).

What we rarely consider to be examples of inflammation are things like insulin resistance, heart disease, cancer, and neurological disorders. We rarely think of mood disorders, cognitive dysfunction, and sleep disorders as being connected with inflammation either. And yet, all of these things have a connection with inflammation. In fact, emerging theories of disease point to the possibility that inflammation may be at the heart of many problems. While I'm certainly not suggesting that all cancer or all sleep disorders are solely caused by inflammation, it is entirely possible that a reduction in inflammation may reduce symptoms. In some cases, it is possible that eliminating chronic, dysfunctional inflammation may reverse a condition.

I am not an expert on all the molecular elements involved in chronic inflammation. However, it is my understanding that the over-expression of inflammatory cytokines such as TNF (also known as TNF-alpha) and IL-6, in particular, are often implicated in chronic inflammation. So herbs that can effectively inhibit these inflammatory cytokines can reduce symptoms and potentially reverse conditions.

Herbs that reduce TNF that are also covered elsewhere in this book include Japanese knotweed (may suppress thyroid function and is estrogenic), turmeric, ashwagandha, milk thistle seed, nettle leaf, reishi, guggul (stimulates thyroid), and gotu kola (stimulates thyroid).

Herbs that reduce IL-6 that are also covered elsewhere in this book include Japanese knotweed (may suppress thyroid function and is estrogenic), turmeric, ashwagandha, schizandra, garlic, and tulsi (remember that tulsi decreases thyroid function).

Of these herbs, two of those that stand out as anti-inflammatory powerhouses are Japanese knotweed and turmeric. Both of these herbs strongly inhibit not only TNF and IL-6, but also nearly every other inflammatory cytokine involved in chronic inflammation. What makes these herbs particularly valuable is that they cross the blood-brain barrier. This means that these two herbs are uniquely suited to address inflammation in the brain, which can be a very real problem that can lead to a host of symptoms that are difficult to diagnose.

Japanese knotweed is my first choice for reducing inflammation, as long as you can tolerate it. This is because it likely has better bioavailability when compared to turmeric. In other words, you can absorb more of this herb more easily.

The downside of Japanese knotweed is that it may suppress thyroid function, and it is estrogenic. However, unless your thyroid is severely compromised, as long as you are otherwise supporting thyroid health, you will likely have no problem with the herb. Exactly how strongly the herb influences sex hormone levels in the body is unclear. So as long as you are not severely estrogen dominant or extremely low in testosterone, then you should be able to tolerate the herb.

The combination of Japanese knotweed and turmeric can be very powerful. Or, if you find that you cannot tolerate Japanese knotweed, then turmeric can be a good substitute. The downside of turmeric is that it is not very bioavailable. Reportedly, taking turmeric with black pepper can greatly increase the bioavailability. However, black pepper is a mild thyroid suppressant, and it can reduce testosterone levels. For most people this should not pose a problem, but if you notice problems, then you may want to leave out the black pepper and see if that resolves the problem. (Note that much turmeric sold as a medicinal herb - at ridiculously high prices considering the price of the raw herb - includes a black pepper derivative called piperine, which is the element from black pepper that is reported to increase turmeric's bioavailability.)

Although I don't know of any evidence that ashwagandha can cross the blood-brain barrier, I believe that it is a good addition to an anti-inflammatory protocol. For one thing, it inhibits major inflammatory cytokines everywhere else in the body apart from the brain. And for another, ashwagandha is reported to strengthen the blood-brain barrier, which can reduce the number of infectious organisms that can cause problems in the brain in the first place.

For inflammation that doesn't fully respond to the aforementioned three herbs, I will also suggest that the addition of the herbs devil's claw, boswellia, and ginger may be helpful.

Reportedly, cannabis can effectively reduce chronic inflammation. However, I would not recommend relying on cannabis as a primary herb for addressing inflammation. My recommendation is to use the aforementioned herbs first to address the inflammation. I feel that cannabis is a very powerful herb that has medicinal value. However, due to the strong potential for habituation, I believe it should be used only for the purposes where it excels and where there are no better alternatives. This preserves the therapeutic potential of cannabis for times of need instead of diminishing the benefits over time because of habituation.

Immune Modulation

One of the important keys to long-term health is to modulate the immune system, and there is a class of herbs that excel at doing exactly that. These herbs are often referred to as tonic herbs or adaptogens.

Adaptogens are safe for daily, long-term use. By definition, they do not produce dramatic effects in moderate doses. However, the results are cumulative, and they work to strengthen and balance the entire body. There are many herbs that fall into this category. There are probably some that grow wild near you, so they need not be exotic herbs. I will share with you some of my favorites as well as some that have been studied in depth.

My personal favorite adaptogen is ashwagandha. This herb is shown to reduce fatigue over time, improve sleep, improve strength, improve mental clarity, relieve depression, and reduce inflammation.

Reishi is a woody mushroom that grows on stumps. I've seen the official species (Ganoderma lucidum) and its close relatives (which I assume have similar medicinal value) growing in New England forests. It is a beautiful mushroom, and it is powerful medicine. Reishi is antiviral and antibacterial. It is anti-inflammatory. It is antioxidant. It improves energy and reduces fatigue over time. It can improve sleep. Reishi does show that it can prevent conversion of testosterone to DHT (which is a more stable androgen), so there is some chance that it could cause an unfavorable sex hormone balance in the body, though this is merely conjecture. Also, it can be a bit drying. The mushroom is revered in Chinese medicine as the mushroom of immortality, and it has a very long history of use.

Rhodiola is an herb that comes from the cold regions of Russia. It effectively reduces depression. It improves mental clarity. It can improve sleep (though it should not be taken close to bed by those who are sensitive), and it gives strength over time.

Cordyceps is another mushroom. It is naturally a parasitic fungus that grows on caterpillars. However, most commercially available cordyceps are grown on rice. Cordyceps is a powerful immune modulator. It also provides important nutrition and sex hormone support.

Eleuthero is another Russian herb, and the Russians have studied it extensively. According to

Russian studies, there isn't anything that eleuthero can't help with. When used in moderate doses long-term, it can reduce stress, reduce fatigue, give strength and endurance, improve mental clarity, and reduce depression.

As I have said, these are just some of the adaptogens that have been best studied and those that I can personally recommend. Remember that these herbs require consistent, persistent use over many weeks or months to begin to receive the full benefits.

Sleep

Sleep is probably one of the most important things we do. It's right up there with eating and loving. Without sleep, you cannot survive for very long. Quality sleep is essential for many aspects of health, including hormonal balance, reducing inflammation, lowering stress, and improving mood, to name but a few.

There are two essential ingredients for successful sleep. First, you need enough sleep, so quantity is essential. And second, you need quality sleep.

Although we are all different, a good rule of thumb is that we need at least 8 hours of sleep every night. Many people shortchange themselves on quantity of sleep. While it may be tempting to cut an hour or two from your nightly sleep in order to accomplish more, in the long term, the studies show that this approach actually reduces productivity. So a better strategy is to commit to enough sleep and learn ways to improve time management and/or priorities.

Now, of course, some of us have found ourselves in the situation in which we block out enough time for sleep, but we find ourselves unable to sleep enough. Either we cannot fall asleep, we cannot stay asleep, or both.

If you find yourself unable to fall asleep, then there may be various reasons for this. One of the most common reasons that people find for why they cannot fall asleep is that their minds are racing, reviewing and planning. If you find yourself in this situation, then you may benefit from practices that give you skills to let go of thinking. See the Stress heading in the Resources section for more on that.

If you find that you are waking in the early morning, unable to fall back asleep, then there may be various reasons for this. Often times, this is linked to cortisol pattern imbalance and/or depleted glycogen stores, which is often the result of diet. People who are eating low carbohydrate diets or calorie-restricted diets, particularly, may find that this happens, so easing up on restrictions in diet can often help with this. There are some studies that show that honey before bed can help with this when it is related to glycogen depletion. Likewise, if you wake up and find you cannot get back to sleep, then a spoonful of honey may help you get back to sleep.

Another reason for this sort of pattern of waking in the morning and being unable to get back to sleep is depleted adrenal function and a general (as in, nonspecific) lack of tonicity or well-being. Again, improving metabolic rate and reducing stress usually can make significant improvements in this regard. However, you may also find that long-term support from adaptogens, such as ashwagandha, eleuthero, rhodiola, reishi, and so forth, improves your sleep over time. This is not a quick fix approach. However, with consistent, moderate doses of adaptogenic herbs, you may see an improvement in your sleep over the course of many months.

Nocturia, or frequent nighttime urination, can be a major cause of reduced quality of sleep. If this is happening to you, then see the Prostate and Urinary Health section.

There are a few herbs that I can recommend that are safe to use as sleeping aids. The first of these herbs is ashwagandha. I recommend taking a larger-than-usual dose of the herb prior to bed to help with sleep. If you are already using ashwagandha as a long-term adaptogen or tonic, then simply use 1 1/2 to 2 times the normal dose just before bed. The traditional way to take ashwagandha before bed is to mix the powdered herb in a small amount of warmed milk. This can be very effective. On the other hand, any form will likely do.

The second herb that I can recommend as a sleeping aid is bacopa. Some people find that they can only use bacopa at night because it always makes them sleepy. I do not notice that effect. However, I do believe that I notice an improvement in the quality of my sleep when I take bacopa before bed. I find that it is best to keep the dose on the lower side since I do notice that it tends to provoke more vivid dreams. A small amount of increased color and motion in a dream is often pleasant. However, too much can reduce the quality of sleep. So a small amount of bacopa can improve sleep quality. Use only if you do not have hyperthyroid problems.

Finally, even though I haven't had a great deal of experience with skullcap, I have experimented with it and found it to be moderately helpful in improving sleep. However, it is my least favorite of the three herbs I've listed here for this purpose. On the other hand, several other respected herbalists, including Susun Weed, list skullcap as one of their favorite herbs for this purpose.

A few notes about skullcap. First, you must use the fresh herb or a tincture made from the fresh herb only. Dried skullcap rapidly loses potency. Secondly, I wrongly reported in the first version of this book that skullcap suppresses thyroid function. However, I cannot actually find any evidence that this is so, and my minimal experimentation with the herb since that time does not suggest to me that it is suppressive of thyroid function - at least not strongly. Thirdly, unlike ashwagandha and bacopa, I do not recommend using skullcap daily. Skullcap seems best suited to those times when you are unable to fall asleep because of racing thoughts or muscular tension.

Generally, it is best not to rely on herbs to help you get to sleep or remain asleep, simply because the herbs may only mask underlying imbalances rather than address the underlying causes. The exception is when using tonic or adaptogenic herbs such as ashwagandha or bacopa, which are safe for long-term use, improve overall health, and also happen to improve sleep.

There are lots of other herbs that may be effective for getting to sleep and perhaps staying asleep. Some of these herbs may be suitable for short-term use. These herbs include motherwort, lemon balm, passion flower, chamomile, hops, and valerian root. I have cautions about some of these herbs, however.

Motherwort, lemon balm, and valerian root are all thyroid suppressants, and therefore, I strongly caution against using these if you have or suspect that you may have low thyroid function. Passion flower may suppress thyroid function, and so I would suggest caution with this herb too if you have low thyroid function.

Also, as a man, I suggest that you avoid hops as a sleep aid. Although hops have some efficacy as a sleep aid, they also create an unfavorable sex hormone balance in men.

Happy sleeping.

Stress

Stress is one of the biggest problems we face. Rather, I should say that a poor response to stress is one of the biggest problems we face, because in truth, stressful things happen, but our response is what truly matters.

Many things may set us into a habit of a poor response to stress. Sometimes the problem is largely a matter of habit that becomes self-reinforcing and digs us deeper into the stress response over time. In my experience, just about everyone can benefit to some degree by learning skills for letting go of stress. I have included my recommendations under the Stress heading of the Resources section of the book.

Other common causes that I have discovered for stress include poor thyroid health, poor metabolic health, or infection. You can see my recommendations on those subjects under Thyroid, Metabolism, and Antibacterial Herbs, respectively.

It is tempting to want to find an herb that you can take as a drug that will eliminate all unpleasant feeling. Yet in my experience, it simply doesn't work that way (with the possible exception of opium poppy, though I would strongly caution against that). For that reason, I strongly suggest learning skills for letting go of stress, and supporting that with sleep and food as well as using herbs to support overall health, such as thyroid health and taking care of infections.

Yet with all that said, there are herbs that demonstrate a remarkable ability to support the body's capacity to handle stress and to meet life with resiliency. You may want to use these herbs in conjunction with other practices and lifestyle choices. Please note that using these herbs as a means to handle more stress with ineffective lifestyle strategies is a very bad idea, so I strongly recommend that you first put into practice effective strategies for letting go of stress and nourishing your body. Then you can consider using these herbs to further nourish your body.

Eleuthero, an herb that used to be known as Siberian ginseng, has been the subject of extensive studies in Russia and in China, and these studies demonstrate that eleuthero can improve the response to stress. Eleuthero is a true adaptogen, meaning that it is remarkably safe and tends to improve health in every way over time. The key word is "time." Eleuthero requires time to work. Expect six months of consistent, daily use to start to see maximum benefits.

Schizandra berry is another herb that has been the subject of many studies that demonstrate its efficacy in improving the response to stress. Schizandra has a long history of use and is considered something of a panacea in Chinese herbalism.

By now you have probably figured that ashwagandha is a darling of mine, so it will come as little surprise to you that I recommend ashwagandha to support a healthy response to stress. Not only does ashwagandha have a long history of use for reducing stress, it also proves out in studies.

Rhodiola rosea is an herb that is used traditionally in the cold regions of Europe and Asia. Traditional uses include improving stress response, and recent studies support this traditional use.

Oats (straw and seed) are a traditional herb said to improve stress response. Oats do contain various alkaloids that have relaxing effects.

Fresh skullcap (or a tincture made from fresh skullcap) can produce a remarkable short-term relief from stress. However, I don't know of any evidence stating that it is appropriate or useful for long-term stress improvement.

Tulsi, also known as holy basil, is an herb that has a traditional use for reducing stress, and the studies substantiate the traditional use. However, I caution against using tulsi for anyone other than those who are hyperthyroid, because tulsi suppresses thyroid function.

Similarly, motherwort and lemon balm can be useful for short-term stress relief. However, they too suppress thyroid function, and as such, should probably only be used by people with hyperthyroid conditions.

Kava Kava is another herb that is often used to reduce stress. Although it does appear to be very effective in reducing stress in the short term, I don't know of any studies or anecdotal evidence supporting that it reduces stress in the long term. Furthermore, I personally found kava kava to be very unpleasant. It gave me extreme nausea. I realize that some people find it to be wonderful. I did not.

Cannabis is yet another herb that many use to reduce stress. Like kava kava, it can be very effective in reducing stress in the short term. However, I know of no evidence that it is effective in reducing stress in the long term, and both personal and anecdotal evidence suggests the same. While it is certainly a very powerful medicinal herb, I do not believe that cannabis should be a primary herb in reducing stress. Reserve for times of extreme need (i.e. reducing homicidal rage).

Prostate and Urinary Health

Any man who has had difficulties with urinary health knows how important it is to be able to pee in a satisfactory and complete manner without pain, dribbling, discomfort, or a sense of incompleteness. And any man who has found himself getting up multiple times in the night to pee knows that it is more than just a minor inconvenience; it can seriously impact health and well-being.

I have struggled with urinary problems for years, and while I haven't yet seen 100% improvement, I have seen significant positive changes. I have also done rather extensive research into the matter. In this section, we'll look at prostate enlargement, urinary infections, kidney stones, and nourishing a healthy urinary system.

Perhaps the most common cause of urinary problems is stress. Stress hormones like cortisol and aldosterone cause an urge to urinate regardless of how much urine is in the bladder. Therefore, chronic overproduction of stress hormones can lead to frequent urination, particularly frequent urination at night. The most common way in which to solve urinary problems is to improve metabolic health and take other measures to improve a poor stress response. Additionally, if frequent urination at night is a problem, many men may find that a bit of salt and honey before bed will help improve the situation.

One of the next most common causes of urinary difficulties for men is known as benign prostatic hyperplasia (BPH). One theory is that BPH is caused by a build-up of androgens in the prostate. Based on this theory, there are several recommendations that researchers have investigated over the years, assuming that herbs that affect androgen receptors in the prostate and other similar actions may have a beneficial action on BPH.

Saw palmetto berry is one of - if not the most - recommended herbs for treating BPH. The studies on saw palmetto berry are mixed, though many do show positive benefits from the herb on prostate health. Researchers suspect that saw palmetto has an action of blocking 5-alpha reductase, which results in less conversion of testosterone to DHT. If this is true, then it's not clear that saw palmetto would be a good choice for men who already have a deficit of stable androgens (since DHT is the most stable androgen). However, the results with saw palmetto are often quite good for mild to moderate BPH, and it has diuretic properties that can increase urine flow while also being nourishing to the urinary system.

What is not clear about saw palmetto is what other effects it may have, especially in regard to thyroid and metabolic health. Although many herbalists recommend saw palmetto for nourishing the entire endocrine system, including the thyroid, and for nourishing metabolic health, I know of no studies that can verify this claim. The traditional use of saw palmetto for increasing weight paints a confusing picture in terms of what effects the herb may have on thyroid function.

I personally have used saw palmetto with good results over the years, and I have not noticed any unwanted side effects as a result. I did not find that it created any noticeable hormonal effects in terms of thyroid or sex hormones, so I do recommend this herb for BPH and for urinary health in general. However, since there isn't a great deal of research on the herb other than studying its effects on the prostate and hair growth, I would suggest using the herb with some caution for other conditions.

Turmeric has shown some remarkable ability to improve prostate health and reduce inflammation. I know of at least one human study that showed that turmeric improved the quality of life for men with BPH by reducing inflammation and infection as well as reducing symptoms. Whether turmeric alone is a complete solution for BPH is not clear. However, I would consider it to be a good herb for men with prostate troubles.

Stinging nettle is another herb that demonstrates positive effects in treating BPH. Typically, the root of the herb is used for this purpose (and traditionally, the root of the herb is considered a powerful male herb). Though there haven't been a lot of studies on the use of nettle for BPH, the few that have been conducted show significant benefits. I personally find nettle root to be helpful.

The African herb, pygeum, is another herb that shows a great deal of benefit for BPH. The studies for pygeum show that it reduces symptoms, acts as an anti-inflammatory, and blocks prostate growth factors that can result in BPH. Unlike saw palmetto, pygeum is not said to block conversion of testosterone to DHT. I don't know of studies demonstrating the effects that pygeum may have on hormonal health overall.

Reishi is a mushroom that has a very strong 5-alpha reductase inhibitory effect, and there are some studies showing that it can be effective in the treatment of BPH. Reishi has a long history of use, particularly in Chinese herbalism. Generally, it is a well-respected herb. It is, however, unclear how extensive the anti-androgenic properties are, so for men with low androgens, I cannot know what the effects would be. For everyone else, however, this seems to be a very safe and health-promoting herb.

Tribulus terrestris fruits (which are spiny, little seed pods) have a long history of use for improving urinary health, and some studies show that they may be useful in reducing BPH. I have personally found tribulus to be a very helpful herb.

Although the leading theory as to the cause of BPH is excessive DHT binding in the prostate, there are other theories that may be valid. One such theory is that BPH is actually caused by excess estrogen rather than DHT. This theory is supported by the fact that incidences of BPH increase with age as androgen levels normally decline and estrogen levels may increase. Therefore, as an alternative to using herbs that reportedly reduce conversion of testosterone to DHT, you may want to experiment with reducing estrogen levels using approaches described elsewhere in this book.

A final note on the subject of prostate enlargement: One very simple, direct, and potentially powerful non-herbal remedy to prostate enlargement is prostate massage. Perhaps the primary reason that this subject is avoided in most contexts is because, to put it crudely, it involves sticking something up your ass. And, for reasons having to do with hygiene and culture, many men don't like to put anything up there.

However, for those who wish to explore prostate massage, generally the two best options for massage are a finger (to be hygienic, one can use a disposable glove or a condom) or a device specifically designed for prostate massage. The prostate is accessible through the rectum on the underside. To get the strongest massaging action you can use one finger (or device) through the rectum and another externally on the perineum. This will gently squeeze the prostate. Prostate massage has been shown to be an effective stand-alone or adjunct treatment to BPH.

Other urinary problems can be caused by an infection of the urinary system, which may include the kidneys, bladder, prostate, or any part of the system. Herbalist Stephen Buhner recommends using a combination of uva ursi, a berberine herb (such as Oregon grape root or barberry), and a tincture of the fresh leaves of bidens pilosa for treating a urinary mycoplasma infection. Mycoplasma is reportedly one of the hardest types of infections to treat, so this combination should be quite effective in addressing most types of urinary infections. Herbalist Susun Weed suggests combining with yarrow. Combined with juniper berries, I think this would address most any urinary infection.

Frankly, I have used uva ursi alone with some good success, and that would be my first approach. There are few herbal suppliers of bidens tinctures (some other species of bidens can substitute for bidens pilosa), so I would start with uva ursi because it is more widely available. If uva ursi alone doesn't do it, then I'd add yarrow. Then, if necessary, I'd add bidens. Then, Oregon grape root or barberry root, if necessary. And finally juniper, if necessary.

In small to moderate doses, all of these herbs should be safe to use over a few weeks or possibly even months. Some herbalists caution against using uva ursi longer than a few weeks, however, so if you want to be cautious, then you should limit uva ursi to a few weeks. I don't recommend using any of these herbs except as necessary since they are fairly strong (apart from bidens, which seems safe for long-term use in tincture form - the fresh leaves can be problematic when used over a long time). I believe that used as necessary up to a few months in moderate doses, these herbs should pose no problem.

Of course, not all urinary problems are caused by BPH or an overt urinary infection. While some of the herbs for BPH are helpful for urinary health more generally (such as saw palmetto and tribulus), there are other herbs that are useful for urinary health apart from prostate concerns.

Corn is reported to be a good herb for men, and the silk from corn is a traditional herb for urinary health. There are several studies that substantiate the traditional use of cornsilk for urinary health, so when you grow or buy fresh corn, don't toss the silk! Eat it.

Goldenrod is an herb that has a history of traditional use as a male herb specific for the urinary system. Goldenrod grows so abundantly in the wild that there is little profit in it, and therefore, there aren't many studies on the herb. The few studies that have been conducted, however, do generally substantiate the traditional use. I include goldenrod here because it is an herb that grows in many places, and you may well be able to find it near you. In New England where I used to live, goldenrod flourishes in the fields. Even here in New Mexico, I have seen goldenrod growing next to the stream that runs past my home. If you can find goldenrod growing wild in a place without any pesticides or toxins, then pick it, infuse it, and drink it. The flowers and leaves are the parts that are traditionally used. Goldenrod is very safe, though some few people get contact dermatitis. If you are one, then you may find it best to avoid the herb.

Yarrow is another herb that may help prostate and urinary health. Although I know of no studies substantiating this use, I do know of some anecdotal evidence that it can help. Yarrow is both antibacterial and anti-inflammatory, and because yarrow grows just about everywhere, it is another good candidate for wild harvesting. Like any plant that you wild harvest, find yarrow in natural places, away from toxins.

Another urinary condition that some of us experience in our lives is kidney stones. I have personally experienced kidney stones twice, and those were the two most physically painful experiences of my life. I turned to herbs to help me through the experiences, and I was surprised by what I found.

There are many herbs that are touted as helping with kidney stones, and most of them did nothing for me. I tried chanca piedra, crampbark, and hydrangea. The truth is that I may not have used enough of them (meaning large enough doses), as there are studies validating that chanca piedra and hydrangea can be very effective in breaking up and eliminating stones. These are herbs worth trying to see if they may work for you.

What finally worked for me on both occasions was to eat large amounts of watermelon. Within hours, the unbelievable pain subsided, and the stones apparently dissolved as my urine became cloudy. Frankly, after writhing in pain, barely able to sleep for several days, watermelon was nothing short of a miracle.

Reportedly, some people have similar experiences to my watermelon experience from cucumbers, lemon, or lime.

Kidney stones can be of several different sorts. The most common sort are said to be calcium oxalate stones, which form when oxalates combine with minerals in the kidneys. Reportedly, reducing dietary oxalates may help if one is prone to oxalate stones, which would mean eating less kale, spinach, chard, celery, and other high oxalate foods. However, I find this hypothesis to be suspect. It may be true, but I'm not convinced. Supposedly, eating calcium-containing foods with high oxalate foods can help by binding the oxalates in the digestive tract instead of absorbing them. Mostly, it seems that the largest factor that may account for oxalate stones is impaired digestion, particularly intestinal problems, so improving metabolic rate and letting go of stress are probably two of the biggest factors involved in reducing the likelihood of oxalate stones. Also, remaining hydrated by drinking fluids that contain both electrolytes (salts) and sugars is helpful. (Note that water, particularly demineralized water, can worsen dehydration because it is not assimilable.)

As many as 15% of kidney stones are reported to be composed of ammonium magnesium phosphate. These types of stones are thought to be caused by a bacterial infection. If you develop these types of stones, then it would seem prudent to address the infection. The common bacteria that are associated with these types of stones are proteus and morganella species. These should respond to a combination of systemic antibacterial herbs (see Antibacterial Herbs for more information), as well as juniper berries, usnea, and honey. While addressing the infection will not resolve the current stones, it should keep new stones from forming. In addition to addressing the infection, you may find that some of the other recommendations in this section are helpful for easing the pain and helping to break up and pass the existing stones.

Uric acid stones account for as many as 10% of kidney stones. These are generally linked to digestive problems - again, mostly intestinal problems.

I have a theory that oxalate and uric acid stones may be caused by a combination of stress and lowered metabolic rate. These two factors contribute greatly to impaired digestion and could account for the link between impaired digestion and stone formation. If I am correct about this, then perhaps the best prevention for kidney stones is to let go of stress and to support metabolic function. Obviously, I offer some suggestions in this book on these subjects under the Stress and Metabolism sections.

If you find that you are prone to kidney stones, then I suggest the following: First, if possible, determine the type of stones. If they are stones formed through bacterial infection, then address the bacterial infection. If metabolic rate is low, then work to improve metabolic rate. Then use herbs to help nourish and cleanse the urinary system. There is good evidence that suggests that chanca piedra and hydrangea may be helpful for this purpose. These herbs would need to be used consistently for weeks or months to see these benefits, though. There's some unsubstantiated talk that hydrangea roots of the species most commonly used for herbal medicine may contain cyanide, which would make it unsuitable for long-term use. I cannot find any proof of this claim, however. It seems that this claim may stem from the fact that some species of hydrangea contain cyanide in the leaves, and because, reportedly, smoking these leaves produces a high, there is some reason to be concerned about the cyanide in the leaves. So if you want to be on the safe side, then use chanca piedra, also known as bhumyamalaki (the Latin name is Phyllanthus niruri or amarus - same plant).

I would also recommend some of the other herbs mentioned earlier in this section that are all-purpose urinary support herbs, such as cornsilk, goldenrod, nettle root, and tribulus terrestris.

Horsetail is another herb that is traditionally used for urinary health, though I have never used it long-term.

Hair Health

There are many reasons that men may lose hair. The most common reasons of which I am aware for hair loss in men are stress, lowered metabolic rate, poor thyroid health, infection, and so-called androgenic alopecia (or male pattern baldness).

At present, I happen to have a thick head of hair. Several years ago I was very, very sick. I was stressed and my metabolic rate was extremely low. At that point, I started losing hair in clumps. Since then, I have discovered effective ways to let go of stress, I have vastly improved my metabolic rate, and my hair has become thick and healthy once again.

If you are losing hair and you are stressed and/or you have a low metabolic rate, then I encourage you to look to the Stress and Metabolism sections of the book for some insights on how you may go about improving those conditions. You will likely find that this is the best first step in addressing this type of hair loss.

Likewise, if you are losing hair and you have a known thyroid disorder, then I suggest that addressing thyroid health is likely the best approach to the hair loss.

If you are losing hair and you have a known infection, then addressing the infection is a logical first step.

Inflammation is also implicated in hair loss, including androgenic alopecia. Specifically, the over-expression of the cytokine known as IL-1beta may be involved, so herbs that reduce IL-1beta may be helpful in slowing or reversing hair loss. Herbs that inhibit IL-1beta include ashwagandha, turmeric, nettle leaf, schizandra, guggul, and reishi.

If you believe that you are losing hair due to androgenic alopecia, then I will offer you some insights that may be of value to you. I must preface this by saying that, to the best of my knowledge, I have never personally experienced androgenic alopecia, so what I share with you in this regard is anecdotal for the most part.

Before I share with you possible ways to address so-called pattern baldness, I want to share a few words about attitude and expectations. Although I have never experienced pattern baldness, I have experienced some other things related to physical appearance that have given me insights into the insecurities and fears that can arise from something such as pattern baldness. In my case, I developed breasts as a boy, and they remained with me until the present day. (I have written another book on this subject.) I obsessed about this for decades, and I was miserable and insecure about it. Eventually, I came to realize that there's actually nothing wrong with that. It's my body. It looks the way it does. And I actually find that when I am happy with my body, then other people are too.

So while there is some possibility that herbs and lifestyle changes may reverse hair loss, they may not. Either way, consider that learning to accept your body as it is can only be helpful. Baldness isn't inherently a bad thing. It doesn't mean anything bad about you, and many people may find a bald head to be very attractive.

I know of one author, Danny Roddy, who believes that so-called androgenic alopecia is actually a metabolic problem rather than a hormonal problem. It is very difficult to know if he is correct about that. I suspect that he may be right in some cases and wrong in other cases. However, because he and perhaps others have benefitted from taking a metabolic approach to hair loss, then I once again encourage you to consider if low metabolism may be a factor for you.

There are several mainstream theories about pattern baldness, though the most prominent is that high levels of free androgens (though low overall levels of androgens) coupled with high levels of 5-

alpha reductase result in high levels of DHT in the scalp, which results in hair loss. (Note the similarity between the theory of pattern baldness and the theory of BPH.) This, of course, begs the question of why this would be so. And, of course, metabolic dysfunction could be a contributor, as could stress, as could lots of other things.

If the theory is correct that high levels of unbound androgens and high levels of 5-alpha-reductase contribute to pattern baldness, then it is reasonable that herbs that address these issues may help reverse hair loss.

The herbs that are conventionally used to help reverse hair loss include saw palmetto, pygeum, and nettle root. The studies testing the efficacy of these herbs for reversing hair loss have been limited and inconclusive. However, the results so far have been encouraging.

I'll also offer you some tips for general hair care.

The natural pH of the scalp and hair is acidic in a range from 4.5-5.5. If you use products on your head that are either too acidic or not acidic enough, then you can damage hair and create problems for your scalp.

The easiest way to test pH is to use pH strips that are available in most pharmacies, many health food stores, and online. Most shampoos are not pH balanced. Plus, they usually contain lots of chemical additives that can harm hair. So generally, if you are concerned about your hair health, then you may want to reconsider using commercial hair products.

Instead, you can use an herbal hair rinse to wash your hair instead of harsh shampoos. One of the most popular herbs for use in an herbal hair rinse is soap nuts since they have natural cleansing properties and have a good pH level. In addition, some people find that the following herbs are helpful additions to hair rinses because they add various properties that can be beneficial for hair: rosemary, amalaki, and horsetail.

Massaging the head with an herbal oil is also a traditional practice that studies show has benefits for hair health and hair growth. Some of the best oils are coconut, sesame, and olive, as well as the more exotic jojoba oil. These oils can be infused with herbs to offer more benefits. The ayurvedic herb, bringaraj (eclipta alba), has a long tradition as an herb for hair health. Although I know of no human studies, the animal studies bear out the traditional use of the herb. The herb rosemary is another herb that has a long tradition as a hair herb that has some recent studies substantiating the traditional use.

Hair Recipes

Here are two recipes for hair care products. The first is a massage oil for nourishing the scalp and hair. The second is a gentle hair rinse that can be used to wash hair in place of chemical shampoos.

Ingredients:
- 1 cup olive oil
- 4 tbsp bringaraj
- 8 drops 100% pure rosemary essential oil

Mix all ingredients in a glass jar with a sealing lid. Place somewhere to let it infuse for at least two weeks. Shake daily.

After two weeks, strain the bhringaraj powder from the oil using a fine mesh strainer, cheesecloth, or fabric.

Store the oil in a jar, and use small amounts to gently massage your scalp at least once a week.

Ingredients:
- 4 soap nuts
- 2 tbsp nettle leaf
- 1 tbsp rosemary
- 1 tbsp ginkgo
- 1 tbsp saw palmetto

Mix all the ingredients with 2 cups of boiling water in a glass jar with a lid. Let it sit for 8 to 24 hours. Then strain the plant material. You can save the soap nuts to reuse them up to 5 times (or maybe even more).

Use this hair rinse in place of shampoo. Use about half a cup per wash. Store the rest in the refrigerator where it will keep for a few days.

When you use this rinse, slowly pour it on your scalp, and massage it into your scalp and hair. It will not lather nearly as much as shampoo. However, it is very effective, and it is better pH balanced than most shampoos. Leave the rinse on your scalp and hair, massaging gently for about 5 minutes. Then rinse.

Insulin

Insulin is a hormone that gets a lot of attention in the public light these days. Insulin is the hormone that shuttles glucose into cells, however, due to various problems, this may not happen. The results can range from mild to life-threatening.

Insulin is made in the pancreas. In some cases, the pancreas is unable to secrete enough insulin, which results in what is known as type 1 diabetes.

Even when the pancreas does secrete enough insulin, it is still possible for complications with insulin to arise. This is usually because of what is known as "insulin resistance." Insulin resistance means that cells cease to be properly sensitive to insulin, so even though there is enough insulin, the cells aren't getting the energy they need. Because the insulin isn't being picked up by the cells, it ends up in other parts of the body where it can cause problems. The theory is that eventually insulin resistance can lead to type 2 diabetes.

Honestly, I do not know of any solid evidence of herbs reversing type 1 diabetes. There are some anecdotes of various herbs being used to improve pancreatic function and reverse the condition. However, I know of no studies demonstrating that herbs (or anything else) can consistently reverse the condition. There are some preliminary studies that demonstrate that turmeric may play a role in improving pancreatic function. Berberine-containing herbs, such as goldenseal, Oregon grape, and barberry, also show the ability to slow or halt the progression of the condition.

When it comes to insulin resistance, however, there is quite a lot of evidence now that herbs can improve or even reverse the condition entirely.

The alkaloid berberine, which is contained in many herbs around the world (goldenseal, Oregon grape, and barberry are some of the most common western herbs containing berberine), has been the subject of a fair number of studies now. The studies demonstrate that berberine is at least as effective as the leading antidiabetic drug, metformin, in reducing blood glucose levels. However, what makes berberine herbs really exciting is that they not only reduce blood glucose, but they can improve insulin sensitivity. If you choose to use berberine herbs to help with insulin resistance and you are currently taking antidiabetic drugs, then you should be careful to monitor blood sugar and adjust drug doses accordingly. And, of course, in that case you should work with your doctor to make necessary adjustments.

Fenugreek has also demonstrated the ability to improve insulin sensitivity. Human studies showed that fenugreek improved fasting glucose levels over eight weeks. When fenugreek is added to food, it can produce glucose levels following the meal. I recommend small amounts of fenugreek added to food or taken in a capsule with meals.

Cinnamon is yet another herb that when combined with food can improve the glycemic response, which can be very helpful for those who have insulin resistance. I recommend small amounts of cinnamon added to food or taken in a capsule with meals. Cinnamon added to hot water, milk, or apple juice is an enjoyable beverage as well.

With herbs taken as food, such as fenugreek and cinnamon, I believe it is best to eat these herbs on a rotation and only in small amounts. More is not always better.

Resistant starch, which is found in foods such as raw potatoes and raw tapioca, also can improve insulin sensitivity. There are several studies that demonstrate that resistant starch shows improvements in insulin sensitivity in humans with type 2 diabetes. Resistant starch must be raw because it breaks down at 160 degrees Fahrenheit. So raw potatoes are the most convenient source. Otherwise, unmodified potato or tapioca starch is an option.

Also, insulin resistance is now connected with an over-expression of several inflammatory cytokines - specifically TNF (also known as TNF-alpha) and IL-6 - so herbs that inhibit TNF and IL-6 may improve insulin sensitivity, either reducing symptoms or perhaps even reversing insulin resistance. See the Reducing Inflammation section for lists of herbs.

Antibacterial Herbs

I use the term "antibacterial" here simply because it seems like the clearest way to describe the particular way in which these herbs may be used, which is to eliminate infections of pathogenic bacteria.

Much of what I share with you in this section is informed by an excellent book, Herbal Antibiotics by Stephen Buhner. Though I have personal experience with all the herbs that I share with you in this section, I find that Buhner has done some impressive research and brought together insights and information regarding the use of herbs to address infections.

Broadly speaking, herbs (and any other substance) are either restricted in their action to particular parts of the body, or they are able to cross into the blood. I like Buhner's simple terminology, and so I will keep it for this discussion. He refers to those herbs that can cross into the blood as systemics and those that remain restricted as non-systemics.

Buhner suggests that most herbs are restricted to the skin, the digestive system, or the organs through which they are eliminated (such as kidneys or lungs). Theoretically, then, all herbs should be effective within the digestive system. And if an herb is eliminated through a particular organ, then we usually say that the herb has an affinity for that organ. For example, juniper is traditionally considered to have an affinity for the urinary system, and it turns out that juniper is excreted largely through the kidneys.

Systemic herbs have the broadest reach. If an infection is truly systemic, then a systemic herb is the ideal candidate for treating the infection. If an infection is not systemic, however, then using non-systemic herbs is often more appropriate. So, for example, if an infection is apparently limited to the kidneys or bladder, then juniper may be a great candidate. Sometimes it is necessary to use both a systemic and a non-systemic herb in combination to see satisfactory results.

There are many systemic antibacterial herbs. However, two that I have learned about from Stephen Buhner's work that I have seen work miracles are sida acuta and cryptolepis. My sister had a bout of pneumonia that was worsening for several weeks. I got her tinctures of these two herbs, and within days she was feeling great. I have personally used these herbs for infections, including long-standing post-nasal drip with very good results.

A third that I also learned about from Buhner's work is an herb called bidens (Bidens pilosa is the primary species that has been researched, though several other bidens species are likely interchangeable). This herb is a systemic antibacterial as well. It has a particular affinity for the urinary system, however, and I can attest that it is quite wonderful for addressing urinary infections, which is the main reason I mention it here. However, it also is active against a variety of bacteria systemically.

For systemic antibacterial herbs, the first two are my favorites. They are exotics. Both of them grow in tropical regions, so they must be imported at this time (though I am hoping to experiment with growing them myself). Normally, I have a preference for plants that grow locally. However, these two herbs are so impressive thus far that I do not know of substitutes for systemic infections.

For additional systemic antibacterial support, I like bidens, particularly if there is a urinary component.

For non-systemic antibacterial herbs, my favorites are as follows: For infections of the digestive system, liver, or mucous membranes, I like Oregon grape root or barberry root. For infections of the urinary system, I like juniper berries and uva ursi. For skin or respiratory infections, I like usnea. However, these herbs can often be combined for good effect. Even though usnea seems to have an affinity for the respiratory system, this doesn't mean that it doesn't also have some benefit for the urinary system or the digestive system, for example.

I highly recommend Stephen Buhner's Herbal Antibiotics Second Edition as a very impressive resource for antibacterial herbs and their uses. In the book, he gives detailed descriptions of the herbs and their uses, and he gives recommendations for specific types of infections.

Liver

The liver, like all of the organs of the body, is remarkably complex. It plays a critical role in many processes within the body. For example, the liver produces many hormones, helps with digestion, metabolizes wastes and toxins, stores energy, and synthesizes proteins.

Diseases and dysfunction of the liver is not uncommon. Although I doubt that they are as rampant as many dubious "cleanse" product manufactures would like us to believe, nonetheless, there are plenty of good reasons to nourish and care for the liver in a balanced and natural way. If you find yourself with liver dysfunction, then it is particularly important to care for the liver.

Some of the most common liver dysfunctions are thought to be caused by viral hepatitis infections, alcohol damage, so-called fatty liver disease, and various drugs (both prescription and nonprescription).

The wonderful news is that the liver is also said to have amazing regenerative capacity. As such, when you nourish and care for your liver, you may see significant improvements.

There are many herbs that can help with detoxifying and maintaining a healthy liver. However, before we talk about those herbs, I'd like to first discuss some of the important lifestyle factors that play an important role in liver health. If you violate some of the basic needs of the liver, then all the herbs in the world may not be able to do enough to keep your liver healthy.

By and large, it would seem that the liver can function within a wide range of parameters, so there is no need to be absolutely rigid in doing everything "perfectly" in order to keep your liver healthy. However, following some guidelines for most of the time can make a big difference in how healthy your liver is.

One of the roles that the liver plays is detoxification. Many toxins are metabolized and then excreted by the liver, so the fewer toxins you are exposed to, the less work your liver has to do in this regard. Conversely, the more toxins you are exposed to, the more taxing it is on your liver, so minimizing toxins is a great way to help your liver.

Some of the common ways that modern humans are exposed to toxins are through chemicals on and in food, using or being exposed to pesticides, chemicals in the home, chemical body care products, drugs, and water. Therefore, if you believe that your liver may be burdened, then it is sensible to give preference to foods produced without chemicals, such as pesticides. It is sensible to avoid using pesticides or frequenting locations in which pesticides are used. You may want to reduce chemicals in the home, including chemical cleaners, synthetic fragrances, and chemically-treated furniture. You may want to switch to using body care products (soaps, shampoos, etc.) that have only natural and nontoxic ingredients. Minimize drug use to whatever extent possible - for this you may need to consult with a medical professional. And if your water is treated municipal water, then you may want to at least run the water through a carbon filter to reduce toxins.

Another way in which the liver can be burdened and harmed is through excessive alcohol consumption. For most people, moderate amounts of alcohol seem to be just fine. However, excessive alcohol consumption is closely linked with liver disease and cirrhosis. So if you drink excessively, then find ways to reduce your alcohol consumption. If alcohol is your way of unwinding or numbing yourself to stress, then finding other ways to let go of stress can help you doubly, because it can reduce the amount of alcohol you consume and it can unburden your liver of stress, which is another major contributor to liver problems. See the Stress section in the Resources section of the book for specific suggestions.

There is no shortage of dietary advice for helping the liver available in books, on the internet, from well-meaning friends, and elsewhere. Much of the advice is extreme - suggesting greatly reducing or eliminating fats, sugars, cholesterol, and other foods. However, in actual human studies, the results suggest that much of this advice may be misguided. It seems that the liver needs a few things to function (apart from a reduction in toxins and alcohol). Those things include enough energy, B vitamins, fat-soluble vitamins, quality protein, and choline. Practically speaking, this makes liver (as in beef liver or lamb liver) the ideal food for liver health since animal liver contains (not surprisingly) all of these necessary nutrients. Eating liver once every week or two can be a great boon to liver health. Otherwise, making sure to eat nutrient-dense foods, including whole dairy, egg yolks, and gelatin-rich meats, is a good way to get these nutrients.

Once you are supporting your liver with sensible lifestyle and dietary practices, then it is worthwhile to consider what herbs can further support optimal liver health.

There are a great many herbs that are helpful for the liver. Some of the easy-to-find superstars are as follows:

Dandelion - yes, the humble dandelion - is an amazing herb for the liver. The leaves, flowers, and roots are all good for the liver, though the roots are the part traditionally used for this purpose. Not only is dandelion a traditional liver herb, but recent studies substantiate the traditional use. Since dandelions grow just about everywhere, you probably won't have a difficult time finding them. Of course, it is very important that you collect dandelions from non-toxic locations, so don't collect them from city lots, near roadways, chemically-treated lawns or fields, or other such locations.

Turmeric is perhaps best known as the spice that gives Indian curries their orange color and distinctive taste, and quite a few studies now demonstrate what herbalists have long known, which is that turmeric is healing for the liver.

Thistles are traditionally used to support liver health. While any part of the thistle can be used for this purpose, the seeds of the milk thistle plant are the most studied parts of the plant for liver health. Although the studies are mixed, generally, the results are favorable in support of using milk thistle seeds for liver health. I have seen some rather remarkable results in a few cases where people started eating a small amount of ground-up milk thistle seeds every day.

These three herbs I've already mentioned are my favorites. I believe that using these herbs regularly is usually enough to support liver health for most people. However, I will include two more herbs here for supporting liver health in specialized situations.

First, for any potential liver problems that either don't respond fully with the first three herbs or that you suspect may involve an infection of the liver, either Oregon grape root or barberry root can be valuable.

Finally, if you feel that your liver is "stagnant," meaning that things aren't moving as they should, then you can use small doses of yellow dock root. Although some herbalists (such as Susun Weed) feel that yellow dock root is a nourishing tonic suitable for daily use, I find that it is a strong herb with laxative properties that is best reserved for times of need and used in relatively small doses. The laxative properties are very weak compared to herbs with laxative reputations. However, do not make the mistake of using too much yellow dock root.

Sex

There are a lot of herbs marketed to men as boosting sexual appetite, erection strength, potency, and so forth, and I find that this is largely unconscionable. While some (few) of the herbs may well be very effective for the purpose for which they are marketed, they often come with unwanted side effects. Others are ineffective. And the majority of them may be helpful, but in subtle ways over the long term rather than the ways in which they are marketed.

To begin with, I think it is important to point out that our culture may set our expectations in unreasonable ways. It is my personal experience that having an insatiable sexual appetite can be very unpleasant, so I caution that aiming for this may be counterproductive to living a happy and satisfying life.

Rather, I believe that when metabolism and hormonal health are optimal, then a man will have a greater likelihood of having a satisfying sexual life. Balance seems to be the key. Desiring sex all the time is probably imbalanced (though to each their own). On the other hand, having the physical capacity to enjoy satisfying sex when the situation naturally presents itself is important.

My intention in this section is to offer you insights on how you can balance your health to support a satisfying sexual experience. To me, this means that you aren't obsessing over sex day in and day out. Rather, you are capable of having satisfying sexual experiences on a daily, weekly, or monthly basis in a way that is appropriate for you and your sexual partner(s).

Although there is no rule, there does seem to be a correlation between spontaneous erections during the night and morning (known as nocturnal penile tumescence, or NPT) and health. So if you do not experience these spontaneous erections, particularly noticeable during the morning before getting out of bed, then this may be an indicator of imbalance.

Many men find that lowered metabolic rate and stress are two likely causes of decreased or absent NPT. Both lowered metabolic rate and stress are causes of hormonal imbalance, particularly reduction in androgen levels, so resolving these issues often can be remarkably helpful in improving sexual health. I can attest personally that as my metabolic rate decreased over the years and my stress levels increased over the years, my sexual health dramatically decreased. However, upon consistently eating enough and learning to let go of stress, my sexual health dramatically improved. So I am a believer that these two factors can play a huge role in sexual health.

Always, my first recommendation is to consider the role that metabolic and hormonal health may be playing in sexual health.

Secondly, consider your overall urinary health. If you are experiencing symptoms of BPH or other urinary disorders, then look to the Prostate and Urinary Health section for some ideas about how to make improvements

If you are otherwise fairly healthy and yet you experience sexual difficulties, then there is one other factor that may be worth considering prior to looking to herbs for help. There is some evidence that suggests that overstimulation (psychologically, that is), particularly through the habitual use of pornography, can create a psychological condition that can cause sexual dysfunction. If you find yourself in this situation, then reportedly, simply leaving off the pornography for some time can reset the nervous system and resolve the problem.

Now, if you want to use herbs to support your sexual health, then I will give you my top picks.

There are lots of aphrodisiac herbs that are stimulating. Some, such as yohimbe, are extremely stimulating, and can even be potentially dangerous. Others, such as the Amazonian herbs catuaba and muira puama, are stimulating in a safer way, though still, I question whether these herbs are really necessary for most men. If you want to use these herbs, then I recommend catuaba and muira puama as some of the safest sexual stimulants. I would recommend avoiding yohimbe. Even the popular herb epimedium (also known as horny goat weed) is not one that I really endorse. Though it is relatively safe, I haven't personally found it to be valuable as a sex aid (though undoubtedly it is a valuable herb in other respects).

If you want herbs that can offer short-term aphrodisiac properties and functional support for erectile strength, then I recommend that probably the two safest herbs for this are fenugreek and ginkgo.

Mostly, I encourage using herbs that offer long-term nourishment of the male sexual system. My top herbs for this purpose are ashwagandha, tribulus, and nettle root. I believe that these three herbs offer superb nourishment and support of the male sexual system and the body overall.

Otherwise, don't be taken in by marketing hype. There are no herbs that are going to increase the size of your penis in the long term. While there are some stimulant herbs that can potentially increase sexual desire and/or erection frequency and strength, many of them are unnecessary when overall health is optimal. Some can even be dangerous or have unpleasant side effects.

A Man's Herbal Guide

Using Herbs

In what follows, I profile some of my favorite herbs and the herbs that I personally have used and found to be beneficial. I strongly encourage you to test herbs before using large amounts of them. Everyone responds differently and ends up having a different relationship to various herbs. What works for one will not always work for another. Though the herbs that I recommend are generally very safe, you still should exercise prudence when getting to know a new herb.

Many of these herbs are safe for regular use. However, I caution against using most herbs daily for long periods without a good reason. Some of these herbs - such as ashwagandha, eleuthero, schizandra, and tribulus - are generally classified as adaptogens, which means that they are considered to be healthy for regular use, improving health consistently over time. Yet, I believe that it is best to use these herbs regularly for periods with intervals of non-use. There is no set schedule for this that will work ideally for everyone, so you can determine what works best for you. It may be one week on and one week off or two weeks on and four days off or any other schedule that works for you. A schedule with intervals of non-use also helps you to judge how the herb may be helping you, hurting you, or unnecessary. Ideally, most of the herbs that you use should help you to restore balance so that you do not need the herbs in the long term. For example, while ashwagandha may help with sleep, ideally it will help you to rediscover the natural balance that allows you to sleep deeply and refreshingly without any herbs.

Finding Herbs

Herbs are plants, not drugs. Even though we may use them as drugs, it is, in my opinion, a mistake to think of them as drugs. I believe this is a mistake for several reasons. For one thing, thinking of herbs as drugs cuts us off from developing relationships with the herbs, discovering the nuances and personalities of the plants and their medicines. For another thing, when we think of herbs as drugs, this puts us in a position where the manufacturer owns the medicine and the process, and we must purchase from them.

Yet because herbs are plants, we have a wonderful opportunity to go directly to the plants. Granted, some of the herbs that I discuss in this book are exotics that do not grow wild where we live or cannot even be cultivated easily where we live. For example, saw palmetto is a tree that grows in subtropical climates. It is native to Florida. Since I do not live in Florida, I cannot find saw palmetto growing wild where I live. Neither can I easily cultivate saw palmetto where I live.

However, many plants do grow wild where I live: dandelion, goldenrod, juniper, yarrow, oak, horsetail, tribulus (I was excited to find that this grows right next to my house!), and usnea, for example. And in many places in North America it is also possible to find hydrangea, barberry, nettle, and milk thistle. If you happen to live in Florida, then you may be able to find saw palmetto.

I believe that wild herbs are usually more potent. Plus, when you wild harvest herbs, you can get them fresh, which is wonderful.

If you wild harvest plants, then do ensure that you have properly identified the plant. While plant identification is outside of the scope of this book, you can find some good regional plant identification guides through various online and offline resources. Also, collect herbs from areas that are clean and haven't been exposed to toxins, such as pesticides. Gather away from roads, industry, and urban areas.

If you do not wish to collect your own herbs or if you wish to use herbs that are not available in your area, then I encourage you to seek out quality herb suppliers. The quality of encapsulated herbs sold in grocery stores, Walmart, and GNC is likely not very good, so I encourage you to find suppliers of very good quality herbs that are either wild harvested or grown organically. I have a list of quality herb suppliers in the Resources section of the book.

Herbal Medicines

You can take herbal medicines in various forms. You can eat fresh herbs. You can eat dried herbs. You can infuse herbs in water. You can infuse herbs in oil. You can extract herbs into alcohol. You can insufflate powdered herbs. You can smoke herbs. You can cook with herbs. You can apply herbs to the skin. There are plenty of ways to use herbal medicines.

How you use a particular herb depends on the herb itself (since different herbs work best in different forms) as well as your preferences. For practical purposes, the most common ways to use herbal medicines internally are:

- tincture - A tincture is an extraction of an herb into a menstruum, which typically involves a combination of water and alcohol. Tinctures are very convenient, they generally are more assimilable than other forms, and they allow for fresh or delicate herbs to be preserved for later use. Not all herbs work well in tincture form, though most do.

- powdered - Dried and powdered herbs may be encapsulated, mixed into food or beverage, or eaten straight. Powdered herbs are nearly as convenient as tinctures, but they lack the shelf life. Most tinctures will last for years, whereas powdered herbs are typically only viable for a few months at best. Also, many herbs simply do not dry well. For example, I have found that herbs such as cleavers or chickweed (neither of which I discuss in this book) are only viable medicine when fresh.

- infused - Herbal teas (or, more accurately, tisanes) are a popular way to use herbal medicine. Dried or fresh herbs can be placed in hot water and allowed to infuse into the water. (Cold infusions are also possible, though less common.) After the herbs have infused, the plant material is strained and the liquid is consumed. While this is often an effective way to use herbal medicines, it is, in my opinion, the least convenient, and so I rarely find myself doing this.

- decocted - A decoction is when herbs are simmered for a long time, creating a concentrated liquid once the plant material is strained. I find that decoctions work best with hearty herbs, such as roots and berries.

Of course, you can invent other ways to use herbs, too. For example, I make herbal jams. I decoct herbs, strain the plant material, and then add enough raw cane sugar so that when it cools, it forms a thick paste. This way, the herbal medicine keeps for a long time, whereas a normal decoction will only keep for a day or two.

In the following herbal profiles, I will share with you the ways in which I find it is best to work with the specific herbs. Of course, you are welcome to experiment on your own.

Ashwagandha

Ashwagandha is a member of the nightshade family, related to famous plants such as tomatoes, potatoes, eggplant, belladonna, and tobacco. The plant has a familiar appearance to anyone who has grown or encountered wild nightshades. And, it does produce little fruits known as winter cherries.

However, it is the root that is traditionally used in herbal medicine. Ashwagandha has a long tradition in Ayurveda, which is the Indian body of knowledge of life and health. The traditional uses of ashwagandha include improving sleep, reducing stress, increasing strength, improving immunity, and improving cognitive function.

There are studies showing that ashwagandha can, in fact, be quite valuable in reducing the negative effects of stress, reducing anxiety, stabilizing blood sugar, improving brain function, increasing memory and learning, modulating thyroid function, and more.

I find that ashwagandha is quite effective as a raw powder, in capsules, and infused or decocted in water or milk. Personally, I have never used a tincture of ashwagandha.

Traditionally, ashwagandha has been used in various ways. Mixing the powdered root with honey and/or butter is traditionally considered to be one of the best ways in which to use the herb. Ashwagandha is also traditionally mixed into milk.

I personally find that powdered root is the easiest and most versatile way to work with the herb. Logically, powdered herbs lose their potency faster than whole herbs, so if you opt for powdered roots, then be sure to use what you have within a few months.

Ashwagandha can help greatly with sleep. Although I have never found that it makes me drowsy, I do find that it helps my sleep. Some people do find that it makes them drowsy, however, so it may be best to try ashwagandha in the evening at first to see how it affects you.

I recommend half a teaspoon of the powdered root mixed with a small amount of milk and a bit of honey as an easy way to take the herb. If you warm the milk slightly, this may be particularly helpful for sleep.

If you find that ashwagandha does not make you drowsy, then you can take half a teaspoon twice or even up to three times a day.

Oregon Grape/Barberry

There are many plants that grow around the world that contain the alkaloid berberine, and they often have very similar effects. The two with which I am most familiar are Oregon grape and barberry. Goldenseal is another popular berberine-containing herb. However, goldenseal is endangered in the wild, and therefore many herbalists suggest using an alternative herb in place of goldenseal. So again, I prefer Oregon grape and barberry.

The roots of these herbs are the most concentrated medicines. They are superb for infections of the digestive system and for liver problems. They also may help to prevent drug resistance in pathogenic bacteria, and they are powerful for improving insulin sensitivity.

I believe they are very powerful medicines, and I value them greatly. I use them, and I have a lot of respect for them.

My opinion is that these herbs are not for long-term use as an antibacterial, which requires substantial doses. Rather, they are best for short-term use to clear up a presenting problem. How long that is will vary from case to case. It could range from a day to a few weeks.

I believe that the precautions regarding limiting use do not apply when using the herb to improve insulin sensitivity. Many herbalists recommend limiting use to no longer than a few weeks at a time.

However, I do not believe this is necessary. The doses required to improve insulin sensitivity are small compared to doses for antibacterial effects, and historically, many herbalists have recommended these herbs as long term tonics in small doses.

The herb can be used powdered, infused, decocted, or in tincture form. Many people find the herb to be unpleasant tasting (it is bitter); therefore, infusions and decoctions are often not great options for most people. Encapsulated powder or tincture is often a more agreeable (and more convenient) option.

If you are using these herbs for antibacterial purposes, then I would suggest starting with 1/2 teaspoon of powdered herb three times a day and modifying as appropriate. Or, if you are using a tincture, then follow the recommendations from the maker of the tincture since strengths may vary. Typically, a dose will be anywhere from 30 to 60 drops three times a day.

If you are using the herbs for insulin resistance, then I suggest that you start with a lower dose than if you were using the herbs for antibacterial purposes. Be sure to monitor your blood glucose, especially if you are using drugs to lower glucose. All the human studies that I can find used a dose of berberine, the isolated alkaloid, rather than the whole herb. Although berberine may be one of the most important constituents for improving insulin sensitivity, I suspect that the whole herb works synergistically. And so it is probably a mistake to dose the whole herb based on the berberine content alone. Therefore, I suggest starting with between 1/8 to 1/4 teaspoon of the powdered herb twice a day about 15 minutes before meals. Or, if you are using a tincture, then use between 1/4 to 1/2 of the recommended dose, and do this twice a day approximately 5 minutes before meals. If you are monitoring your blood glucose, then you should be able to adjust the dosage appropriately over time.

Dandelion

Dandelion is a biennial herb, which means that in the first year it produces no flower (and therefore no seeds), instead storing energy into the root. The second year, it produces a flower and then goes to seed, moving along to the next generation of plants.

The leaves of the plant are suitable for herbal use at any time - during the first or second year - as long as they are green and vital. The root, however, is best during the fall of the first year or early spring of the second year. This is because the energy is stored up during this time. Before this time, the root has less energy, and after this time, the energy shifts into producing a flower and seeds. Honestly, I find that roots are *always* good, but they are probably best during the fall or early spring.

I like the taste of dandelion, though it is bitter. I enjoy eating the roots, and I sometimes eat them like I would eat a raw carrot. The leaves are good in a salad in small amounts, and I include the roots in soups. I recognize, however, that not everyone feels this way about dandelion. If you do not like the taste, then encapsulated dried herb or a tincture of the herb may be more suitable for you.

I don't think there is any reasonable upper limit on dandelion. It is not the sort of herb/food that one is likely to eat in large amounts. I mean, even though I like the taste of dandelion, I find that I am satiated by eating a few leaves or a nice, crispy root.

As far as I know, dandelion is a very safe herb that is generally well-tolerated, so please enjoy finding ways to incorporate dandelion into your diet in small ways.

Turmeric

Turmeric is a plant that produces rhizomes that look not entirely unlike small, orange ginger rhizomes. It is a staple in Indian cooking, which is how most of us know of turmeric. However, it also has a long history of use as a medicinal herb.

Orange and yellow bitter-tasting herbs are often powerful liver herbs. Turmeric is no exception. It is a gentle, yet powerful cleansing herb that helps the entire digestive system, with a special affinity for the liver. It stimulates digestion. It has antibacterial properties. And it protects the liver.

Furthermore, turmeric has anti-inflammatory properties that make it helpful for inflammation in the body. And since it crosses the blood-brain barrier, it is anti-inflammatory for the brain as well.

I believe that turmeric works best as a whole herb rather than an extract. The most common form in which turmeric is available is as a powdered herb. I recommend using the herb in food or encapsulated.

Turmeric, like dandelion, I believe is very safe, and as such, I believe there is no reasonable upper limit. A small amount usually goes a long way, and so it is unlikely that you'll find yourself wanting to eat tablespoons at a time. Rather, half a teaspoon added to food or a few capsules of the powdered herb is sufficient.

Japanese knotweed

I first learned of this herb because I got sick with Lyme disease. This plant was growing all around me, and yet I never really noticed it until a friend of mine brought a stalk and leaves over to help me identify it, telling me that the root is supposed to be helpful for Lyme disease. I went in search of the plant, which was not difficult to find (it is an aggressive invasive in New England, where I lived at the time), but finding it growing somewhere other than immediately alongside a busy roadway was a bit of a challenge.

Eventually, I found some growing off of a tiny dirt road that wasn't much in use. I was too sick at the time to dig, so my partner did the digging. It must have taken an hour to dig up some of the fat, woody roots. And without proper equipment, it was difficult to do much with it, so I ended up chopping off pieces and chewing on them, which I do not recommend. It is astringent and has a not-entirely-pleasant flavor.

My recommendation is to either make or purchase a tincture of the root and use it that way. I presently know of only one source of quality, organically-grown Japanese knotweed, which comes from Healing Spirits Herb Farm (see resources section for more information). For the money, your best bet is to purchase the herb from Healing Spirits and then produce a tincture yourself. Or, you can purchase a quality tincture (made from the herb grown at Healing Spirits) from Woodland Essence.

For treating mild-to-moderate chronic inflammation, use one dropperful 3 times a day, if you can tolerate it. For stronger inflammation you can use more, probably up to 4 droppersful 3 times a day.

I strongly encourage you to start with a much lower dose (10 drops twice a day) and work your way up to larger doses slowly. Although this is a very safe herb, it can be hard for some people to tolerate larger doses. I find that I cannot tolerate a large dose of the herb. It may be a thyroid suppressant (though I think the effects in this regard can be offset with thyroid nourishment and support), and it is estrogenic, though the precise effects in the body are not clear to me. So just go slow, and respect the power of the herb.

If you cannot tolerate large doses of the herb, then I suggest lowering the dose to the maximum that you *can* tolerate (which may be just a drop or two at a time for some people), and combining with turmeric and ashwagandha for an anti-inflammatory combination. Boswellia and nettle leaf may also be helpful.

Juniper

Juniper is a plant that grows as a shrub or tree, depending on the species and location. There are many species worldwide. All parts can be used as herbal medicine, though the berries are most commonly used.

Some species of juniper are toxic and should be avoided. I have yet to find a definitive list of toxic species. Apparently juniperus sabina and juniperus oxycedrus are both toxic. These are native to parts of Europe and are sometimes planted as ornamentals in the United States. I have also read cautions regarding juniperus virginana and juniperus silicicola. If you are uncertain of the species and whether or not it is toxic, then it would be best to avoid it.

I presently live in New Mexico, which is abundant in juniper. If you live somewhere without abundant juniper, then you can use several other evergreen species similarly for antibacterial value. Fir and pine are often used for this purpose, as is cedar. In the case of these other evergreen species, the needles or leaves are commonly used.

As far as I know, however, the urinary benefit of juniper is not shared to the same extent by other evergreen species, so if you want to use juniper to benefit the urinary system then juniper berries are probably your best option.

If you want to wild harvest juniper berries, then you want to pick only the purple berries rather than the green.

Of course, you can simply purchase juniper berries from herbal suppliers.

I have read cautions from most herbalists regarding juniper berries, suggesting that they should only be used for a very short time and avoided by anyone with kidney problems. However, I cannot find any actual basis for this caution. As far as I can tell, there are no such cautions from long-standing traditions. You'll have to make up your own mind on the matter. I have never noticed a problem from the berries.

I do suggest that if you decide to use juniper berries longer-term that you use *small* amounts. I recall reading Stephen Buhner's mention that he has eaten 5 berries a day over a long term without any problems.

Also, I have read cautions that state that if you notice that your urine begins to smell like violets that you should immediately cease using the herb, so watch (or smell, rather) for violet-scented urine, and if you notice that, take it as a sign to stop with juniper.

The berries themselves from some species (notably juniperus communis) taste pretty good, so in this case, the easiest way to take this herbal medicine is to eat a few berries. They are strong medicine, so I recommend eating just a few at a time.

You can also infuse the leaves (which may be needles, depending on the species) of juniper or any of the other species mentioned in hot water and drink that.

If you prefer tincture form, then a tincture of juniper should be effective. I have never personally used a tincture of juniper, however.

Usnea

Usnea is a lichen, which means it is a symbiont of algae and fungus. It grows on trees, and I imagine that just about anyone who has visited a forest, even the pine and juniper forests of New Mexico, has seen usnea growing on trees. One of its names is old man's beard because the growth of the lichen resembles, to some degree, a long beard.

Some wild harvesters maintain an ethic of collecting only usnea that has fallen since their view is that this does not harm viable usnea.

If you cannot or will not wild harvest, then you can purchase usnea from herbal suppliers.

Usnea has antibacterial properties that are effective against a wide spectrum of bacteria. It is a non-systemic antibacterial, and apart from the digestive system, it also has a reputation for being particularly effective in cases of infection in the lungs or urinary system.

Usnea can be used directly on the skin or on wounds for infections. Although it can be infused into water, reportedly, it extracts poorly into water. Generally it is extracted in alcohol and used as a tincture.

Milk Thistle

Milk thistle is a flowering plant that is native to Europe and Asia. However, it grows most everywhere now. Most of us have probably seen milk thistle with its classic purple thistle flowers growing at one point or another.

Milk thistle has a long reputation for being a potent liver-helping herb. The seeds are particularly concentrated in the medicinal value for liver ailments.

In addition to its use as a general liver protectant and restorer, herbalists also use milk thistle for cirrhosis and hepatitis. Milk thistle has demonstrated some capacity to treat mushroom poisoning, which makes it one of the few medicines known that can help in cases of otherwise fatal poisoning. It isn't foolproof, of course, but it can help.

I find that ground milk thistle seeds have a mild, pleasant, slightly nutty flavor. Most people seem to agree, so I generally recommend simply eating small amounts of ground milk thistle seed. Some herb suppliers offer ground seeds. I find that it is convenient to grind them fresh in a coffee grinder, and this is less likely to result in highly oxidized seeds.

There is no reasonable upper limit to how many milk thistle seeds one can eat. You are unlikely to find yourself wanting to eat tablespoons at a time, so adding a teaspoon or so of ground seed to food is a good way to add this herb into your diet.

For those who prefer tinctures, the milk thistle tincture is reportedly effective. I have never used a tincture of milk thistle because I find no need.

Saw Palmetto

I have never seen a saw palmetto tree, though I am led to believe that they are palm trees. They grow mostly in Florida. The berries have a long tradition both as food and as medicine.

The most popular use of saw palmetto today is for BPH. Most of the studies demonstrate that it is very effective for this purpose. A few recent studies suggest that it is *not* effective in reducing BPH symptoms. However, anecdotally, many men, including yours truly, find that saw palmetto is very effective in helping with urinary troubles, including BPH.

Saw palmetto is also promoted as helping with hair growth, particularly in cases of so-called androgenic alopecia. Some studies demonstrate that this may be effective for some people.

Saw palmetto does exhibit some anti-androgenic properties. In fact, some believe that this is how saw palmetto can be effective for treating BPH and helping to regrow hair. What is not clear is how extensive the effects are. I have not personally ever experienced noticeable negative hormonal effects from saw palmetto. Theoretically it may be a risk. Still, some claim that the effects are localized to the scalp and the prostate. I do not know what the case it, so caveat emptor.

Saw palmetto berries have a distinctive and strong flavor that I personally find to be agreeable. I don't know that everyone would like the taste, however. Because I find the taste to be agreeable, I have simply eaten the powdered berries when I have used the herb. (The whole, unpowered, dried berries are impossible to chew. They are nearly rock hard.) If you wish to eat powdered berries, then I suggest starting with 1/2 teaspoon three times a day. I don't believe there is a reasonable upper limit. In fact, reportedly, some traditions have eaten the berries as a food.

If you prefer not to taste the berries, then you can use encapsulated powder.

Tinctures of the herb are reportedly effective. I have never used a tincture of the herb.

Nettle

Stinging nettle is a beautiful (in my opinion) plant that grows just about everywhere. As the name implies, it stings. Some strange people, myself included, actually enjoy the stinging sensation that the plant produces when touched with bare skin, but most decidedly do not like the sensation. The plant has many small hairs that inject substances that produce a sustained stinging sensation on the skin; therefore, when harvesting, you may be advised to wear gloves.

The stinging effect is only present in live plants or plants that have recently been picked. When blended, dried, or cooked, the leaves no longer sting. And, in fact, nettle is a rather delicious vegetable that has a flavor not entirely dissimilar to spinach (in my opinion). Like many of the herbs profiled in this book, there is no reasonable upper limit on how much nettle is safe to eat.

The leaves are rich in minerals and contain some of the same properties as the root in terms of men's health. However, the roots are the traditional part used by men.

The roots of nettle are used to improve urinary health and symptoms of BPH. Studies substantiate the traditional use of the herb for these purposes.

I typically use nettle root either as a cut root that I infuse or decoct, or as a powder that I eat or add to foot. I find that the root has a mild and fairly pleasant earthy flavor. I would recommend at least 1/2 teaspoon of the powdered root three times a day or, if using cut root, 1 teaspoon packed root infused or decocted three times a day.

As with many herbs that are foods, I have never used a tincture of nettle. Theoretically it is an effective way to work with the herb, however, so if that is your preference, then it should work.

Uva ursi

Uva ursi is also known as bearberry, reportedly because bears like to eat the berries. The plant is related to manzanita and has the same bell-shaped flowers. The leaves are the part used medicinally.

Although the herb has traditional use in smoking mixtures, the present medicinal use of uva ursi is primarily for treating urinary infections. The leaves contain an antibacterial substance that is one of the most effective for treating many urinary infections.

I have only used the herb as a hot infusion, though reportedly, it is quite effective as a tincture as well.

Stephen Buhner recommends combining with a berberine herb and bidens. Susun Weed recommends combining with yarrow.

Most herbalists caution against using it for more than a few weeks at a time, though they don't say why. The herb does contain hydroquinone, which is potentially toxic to the liver. Then again, it's also found in beer and coffee. Stephen Buhner suggests that the only caution is for extended regular use (years at a time), because the herb inhibits melanin formation and can cause an eye problem. So the conservative cautions may be unnecessarily conservative, but all the same, I'd keep use to a minimum. Use only as long as necessary - days or weeks at a time, preferably.

Bacopa

Bacopa is a traditional Ayurvedic herb that is said to promote intelligence, and the studies back this up. Bacopa can increase memory, attentiveness, and mental clarity when used consistently for several weeks or months. These cognitive effects take time to begin to be noticeable and measurable, so usually the suggestion is to use bacopa daily for six weeks before expecting to notice improvements in these regards.

Bacopa is also a thyroid stimulant (increasing T4) and can improve sleep. These effects are noticeable immediately.

I have used bacopa on and off over the years, yet it wasn't until recently that I started to use it consistently. I do find that it has noticeable effects when used consistently.

I also find that for thyroid support, it is often best to use bacopa with another herb. Guggul has a strong synergistic effect when used with bacopa to support thyroid health because guggul increases T4 to T3 conversion. However, you should only use this combination if you have low thyroid function.

The taste of bacopa is not really pleasant. In fact, some people would describe it as awful. I find it to be only mildly unpleasant, though I wouldn't want to eat much of it. I prefer to use it as a tincture, which minimizes how much I eat (versus eating a half teaspoon of powdered herb or drinking an infusion). However, some people will prefer encapsulated herb to avoid having to taste it at all.

If you use a tincture, then 1 dropper-full 3 times a day is a good dose for most adults. Some people find that it makes them very sleepy, so I recommend trying it first in the evening rather than on a morning when you have to do something else (like drive to work). And start with a lower dose (10-15 drops) to see how you respond to it since larger doses can cause dreams that are "too" vivid.

Sida Acuta and Cryptolepis

Sida acuta and cryptolepis are entirely different plants. However, I group them together here because I use them for similar purposes. I use these herbs strictly for their antibacterial properties. Although they have traditional uses, they are premium exotic herbs that I can presently only obtain through herbal suppliers, and I pay a lot for them, so I use them sparingly and only for the antibacterial qualities.

I honestly know very little about the herbs other than that they are effective against a large number of pathogenic microorganisms. They appear to be very safe. Furthermore, reportedly, they are effective systemically, which makes them very powerful and important herbs, particularly for drug-resistant organisms.

Cornsilk

The silky threads that grow up out of the tops of the ears of corn are powerful medicine for the urinary system. They seem to have an affinity for the urinary system where they impart soothing, anti-inflammatory properties.

Personally, I like to just eat the silk from fresh corn. It has a pleasant taste and a not-altogether unpleasant texture when fresh. When fresh corn isn't in season (which is most of the year), I opt for dried cornsilk, which I infuse.

Some people find good results from encapsulated cornsilk. I have never tried it that way. And cornsilk is sometimes available as a tincture, which reportedly works well, though I have never tried it that way either.

Tribulus

Tribulus is considered to be an invasive in many places. It is also known by the name "puncture vine" because the small fruits have sharp spikes that are tough enough that they have even been known to puncture a car tire. I can attest that they are painful to step on!

The fruits (which are nearly rock hard) are the part used in herbal medicine. The herb has a long tradition in India where it is considered to be an all-around restorative. However, the herb clearly has an affinity for the urinary system.

Studies show that tribulus is an effective diuretic, though what other effects it may have are not clear. Traditionally, it is held that tribulus is a safe diuretic that nourishes the urinary system and does not deplete the body of potassium and other electrolytes, as do some diuretics.

I very much like tribulus. I infuse or decoct the whole fruits, and I mix the powdered fruits with food. I find the latter to be the most convenient, and the fruits have a mild, nutty flavor that is not unpleasant.

I believe that tribulus is quite safe, so any reasonable amount is likely to be fine. I would suggest that a minimum of 1/2 teaspoon three times a day of powdered fruit or five whole fruits infused three times a day would be a good place to start.

I don't usually see tribulus tinctures. I assume that the herb must not extract well in alcohol, so if infusions, decoctions, or unencapsulated powder is not for you, then I suggest encapsulated powder as an alternative.

Goldenrod

Goldenrod is a perennial herb that grows just about everywhere in North America. Like all herbs, goldenrod has many uses, though the most common use of goldenrod seems to be for urinary conditions. The herb is diuretic, which makes it useful for kidney stones, bladder infections, kidney difficulties, and just about anything having to do with the urinary system.

Chances are you can find goldenrod growing near you (unless you live in a huge city). I was delighted to find a patch of goldenrod growing next to the stream by which I live here in New Mexico. There are many different varieties. The species here in New Mexico is small - less than two feet in height - whereas the species common throughout New England can grow nearly as tall as an adult human. Most of the species are said to have similar properties.

The above-ground parts are what are usually used for herbal medicine. The leaves can be harvested throughout the spring and summer, while the flowers can be collected later in the summer. Personally, I believe the flowers are more potent, but the whole plant is effective.

Reportedly, dried goldenrod is effective for herbal medicine. I have not found it to be so, however, so I personally can only recommend fresh herb, which, as I've suggested, most of us can do in season.

Goldenrod tincture made with fresh herb should be effective. I have never tried it, however.

Yarrow

Yarrow is a beautiful flowering herb that grows just about everywhere in North America. Just looking at yarrow is a healing experience, in my opinion. I love yarrow.

Yarrow's most well-known use is as a wound healer. I have never tested this claim, but supposedly, pressing yarrow against a wound will stop the bleeding. It can be used internally for similar purposes, where it is said to tone the venous system.

Yarrow has many other benefits, many of which come from its action of stimulating circulation and its antibacterial properties. Yarrow can benefit most of the body. However, yarrow has a reputation as a strong herb for the urinary system.

Although the dried herb is reportedly effective, I believe that fresh yarrow is much more potent. You can use any of the above-ground parts. I personally like the flowers.

You can eat the flowers fresh, infuse them in hot water, or apply them to wounds. Otherwise, a tincture of the herb is likely to be effective as well, though I have never used a tincture of this plant.

Conclusion

My sincere hope is that this book has been helpful to you. I believe that herbs can be powerful allies in our discovery of health and balance. As I have also endeavored to share with you throughout the book, I do not believe that herbs are the sole answer to everything, however. I believe that we must also take into account the tremendous importance of metabolic health and hormonal balance. When we strike the right balance, *then* I believe that herbs can offer us huge support in maintaining balance and helping us to enjoy life even more.

Resources

Stress

Hopefully I have impressed upon you the importance of learning skills for letting go of stress. When we hold on to stress, this can adversely affect all of our health. It has very real and detrimental effects on digestion, hormonal balance, metabolism, cognition, sleep, and more.

The following are the programs that I can personally recommend for effective ways to let go of stress. Everyone is different, so what works for one will not necessarily work for another. These are not the only effective programs. These are simply the ones that I can personally endorse since I have tried them and found them to be helpful.

Some of these programs have a financial cost associated with them. In those cases, I encourage you to make the smallest investment possible by purchasing nothing more than a book. In my experience, each of these programs can be effectively learned through writing rather than expensive training programs. Your cost should never be more than $20 for any of these programs.

- Peaceful Possibility - This is a program that I created to share with people what I have personally found to be some of the most effective techniques for letting go of stress that I have ever encountered. This is a completely free video training program with more than three hours of video. There is never any cost associated with this program. I invite you to check it out and see if it is helpful for you. I recommend this program above all others since I honestly have found it to be vastly more effective than anything else. (Of course, I am biased, so your mileage may vary. But since it's free, there's no risk to you.) You can learn more at www.peacefulpossibility.com.
- The Sedona Method - You can learn more about this program at www.sedona.com, and you can either find the book at your library or you can purchase it through a retailer. (The expensive training program is essentially an audiobook version of the same material, so I do not recommend anything other than the book.) The program isn't for everyone. Some people find it to be very effective. Some people find it to be frustrating and ineffective. I believe that when one truly understands it, it is very powerful. However, not everyone fully understands the principle of the

program, which is essentially just to let go of attachments to ideas through a simple process of asking yourself three questions - Could I let it go? Would I let it go? When?

• HeartMath - You can learn more about this program at www.heartmath.com. The essence of this program is a simple process of "breathing in and out of the heart." The organization sells lots of other programs and gadgets and gizmos. I *only* recommend the basic techniques that are described in the book that is available through libraries or book retailers.

• The Work of Byron Katie - You can learn more about this program at www.thework.com. The entire program is described in Byron Katie's book, *Loving What Is*. The process consists of four simple questions followed by what she calls a turnaround. I find that this process is very effective for some things and for some people. Other times it doesn't help.

Sea Vegetables

The only source of certified organic sea vegetables (how they get organic certification, I don't quite understand) in which the company has third party test results of the herbs on the website is Maine Coast Sea Vegetables. The company seems to be run by honest people, and the quality of the herbs they sell is top-notch. I find that the quality of Maine Coast

Sea Vegetables is vastly superior to most other sea vegetables I have purchased.

You can find Maine Coast Sea Vegetables products in most natural food stores, or you can order directly from the company from the website, www.seaveg.com.

Dried Herbs, Fresh Herbs, and Tinctures

For most of us, we will want to purchase herbs rather than wild harvesting them. That is fine. If you wish to purchase herbs from a local store, then you may be able to find some quality herbs at natural food stores in your area. If you purchase encapsulated herbs or dried loose or powdered herbs, then ensure that they are organically grown or ethically wild harvested and that they include no fillers. If you are purchasing tinctures, then I recommend looking for tinctures made with organic and ethically wild harvested ingredients. Herb Pharm is an herbal medicine maker that makes tinctures that can be found in most natural food stores, and I find the quality to be quite good.

Otherwise, the following are my favorite online herb retailers.

- Healing Spirits Herb Farm - www.healingspiritsherbfarm.com is a small herb farm with superb herb quality. All the herbs are certified organic, and they are hand-harvested and solar-dried. The owners of the farm are very nice and obviously put a lot of love into what they do. I highly recommend Healing Spirits.

- Woodland Essence - www.woodlandessence.com is a small herb maker with excellent quality herbal medicines. I select Woodland Essence for sida acuta and cryptolepis because they obviously put a lot of love into what they do, they use certified organic alcohol for tinctures, and they are one of the few retailers selling these herbs.

- Bear Wallow Herbs - www.bearwallowherbs.com is a small, one-woman herb company that makes and sells herbal medicines - mostly tinctures. The quality is top-notch, and she uses certified organic grape or cane alcohol. I have been happy with the quality of the herbs I have purchased from her.

- Pacific Botanicals - www.pacificbotanicals.com sells dried (and some fresh) herbs of high quality. Pacific Botanicals has a huge selection. However, the smallest quantity of a single herb that you can purchase from the company is one pound, so Pacific Botanicals is only suitable for large orders.

- Mountain Rose Herbs - www.mountainroseherbs.com sells dried herbs and various herbal medicines such as tinctures, capsules, oils, and more. The selection is huge, and the quality is generally very good. Plus,

Mountain Rose Herbs sells smaller quantities of bulk herbs, starting with 4 ounces for most herbs.

- Banyan Botanicals - www.banyanbotanicals.com sells Ayurvedic herbs that are certified organic. Many of these herbs are difficult to find elsewhere. Banyan Botanicals is the only supplier of organic bhringaraj of which I am familiar.

Seeds and Plants

For those wanting to grow herbs, I highly recommend Horizon Herbs. The website is www.horizonherbs.com. The selection of seeds and starts is absolutely amazing, including lots of very hard-to-find plants. And, everything from Horizon is produced according to organic certifications. I have grown some beautiful and amazing plants from seeds I purchased from Horizon Herbs.

Get My Future Books FREE

If you enjoyed this book (Hey, if you made it this far it couldn't have been that bad), you'll probably enjoy many of my other books about health and wellness. And you can get all my new releases in health and wellness for free by signing up for my mailing list at www.joeylotthealth.com. It's simple, it's free, and it's totally honest and legitimate. Nothing scammy or spammy or anything else like that (i.e. I won't be trying to sell you The 7 Dirty Underground Top Secret Weird Tricks for Rock Hard Abs or Young Living Oils). It's just about free books for those who appreciate my work, because I appreciate YOU. Simple as that.

Connect With Me

I welcome your questions, comments, and feedback of any kind. Please feel free to email me at joeylott@gmail.com. I am now receiving so many emails that I cannot always reply to every email. I do read them all, and I do my best to reply to as many as possible. For the benefit of others, I may choose to publish my response to your email on my blog or in book format. I will maintain your privacy and anonymity if I choose to publish my response.

One Small Favor

My sincere goal in writing is to share something that may be of value to you. And I endeavor to do so while keeping the costs low for readers. The success of my books and my ability to reach other readers who may benefit from my books depends in large part on having lots of thoughtful, honest reviews written about my work. You would do me a great favor if you would please take a moment to generously write a review of this book at Amazon.com. This will only take a few minutes of your time, and you will be helping me a great deal. I sure would appreciate it.

About the Author

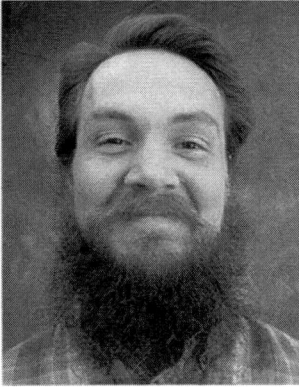

"The secret to happiness is to let go of everything - see through every assumption."

Beginning at a young age Joey Lott experienced intensifying anxiety. For several decades he lived with restrictive eating disorders, obsessions, compulsions, and an inescapable fear. By the time he was 30 years old he was physically sick, emotionally volatile, and mentally obsessed with keeping any and all unwanted thoughts and experiences at bay.

At this time Lott was living on a futon mattress in a tiny cabin in the woods. He was so sick that he could barely move. He was deeply depressed and hopeless. All this despite doing all the "right" things such as years of meditation, yoga, various "perfect" diets, clean air, and pure water.

Just when things were at their most dire, a crack appeared in the conceptual world that had formerly been mistaken for reality. By peering into this crack and underneath all the assumptions that had been unquestioned up to that moment, Lott began a great undoing. The revelation of this undoing is that reality is utterly simple, ever-present, seamless, and indivisible.

Lott's books provide a glimpse into the seamless, simple, and joyous nature of reality, offering a glimpse through the crack in conceptual worlds. Whether writing about the ultimate non-dual nature of reality, eating disorders, stress, disease, or any other subject, he offers the invitation to look at things differently, leaving behind the old, out-grown, painful limitations we have used to bind ourselves in suffering. And then, he welcomes you home to the effortless simplicity of yourself as you are.

Not sure where to begin? Pick up a copy of Lott's most popular book, *You're Trying Too Hard*, which strips away all the concepts that keep us searching for a greater, more spiritual, more peaceful life or self.

13288230R00092

Printed in Great Britain
by Amazon.co.uk, Ltd.,
Marston Gate.